COMPLETE GUIDE

TO

Special Education Transition Services

Ready-to-Use
Help and Materials
for Successful Transitions
from School to Adulthood

Roger Pierangelo, Ph.D. ■ Rochelle Crane, C.S.W.

Library of Congress Cataloging in Publication Data

Pierangelo, Roger.
    Complete guide to special education transition services : ready-to-use
help and materials for successful transitions from school to
adulthood / Roger Pierangelo, Rochelle Crane.
        p.   cm.   .
    Includes bibliographical references.
    ISBN 0–87628–274–5
    1. Handicapped youth—Services for—United States.   2. Handicapped
youth—Vocational education—United States.   3. Vocational guidance
for the handicapped—United States.   4. School-to-work transition—
United States.   5. Parents of handicapped children—United States—
Finance, Personal.   I. Crane, Rochelle.   II. Title.
HV1569.3.Y68P55   1997
371.91—dc21   97–26606
                                                        CIP

© 1997 by The Center for Applied Research in Education

All rights reserved.

Printed in the United States of America

10 9 8 7 6 5 4 3 2 1

ISBN 0-87628-274-5

ATTENTION: CORPORATIONS AND SCHOOLS

The Center for Applied Research in Education books are available at quantity discounts with bulk purchase for educational, business, or sales promotional use. For information, please write to: Prentice Hall Career & Personal Development Special Sales, 240 Frisch Court, Paramus, NJ 07652. Please supply: title of book, ISBN, quantity, how the book will be used, date needed.

**THE CENTER FOR APPLIED RESEARCH
IN EDUCATION**
West Nyack, NY 10994
A Simon & Schuster Company

On the World Wide Web at http://www.phdirect.com

Prentice Hall International (UK) Limited, *London*
Prentice Hall of Australia Pty. Limited, *Sydney*
Prentice Hall Canada, Inc., *Toronto*
Prentice Hall Hispanoamericana, S.A., *Mexico*
Prentice Hall of India Private Limited, *New Delhi*
Prentice Hall of Japan, Inc., *Tokyo*
Simon & Schuster Asia Pte. Ltd., *Singapore*
Editora Prentice Hall do Brasil, Ltda., *Rio de Janeiro*

DEDICATIONS

I dedicate this book and all the work that went into it to my loving wife Jackie and my two beautiful children Jacqueline and Scott; to my parents, who got so much pleasure from being parents; to my sister Carol, who would make any brother proud; and to my brother-in-law Dr. George Giuliani, who throughout our relationship has always been there unconditionally.

Roger Pierangelo

This book is dedicated to my parents, Harry and Rae; to my brother Larry; and to my children, Valerie and Alex, whose support and encouragement have been the foundation of all my accomplishments.

Rochelle Crane

ACKNOWLEDGMENTS

➤ All the students, parents, and teachers of the Herricks Public School District, New Hyde Park, NY, that I have had the pleasure of meeting, knowing, and helping in my twenty-four years in the district.

➤ Rochelle Crane, my coauthor, a good friend and colleague for twenty years. It is not only Rochelle's incredible journey and accomplishments in life that make her a special person but the accomplishments of those whose hearts she has touched. For that, I am forever grateful.

➤ Again, Ollie Simmons, an extraordinary individual and personal friend, who always helps me start the day with a smile.

➤ Helen Firestone, one of the most instrumental individuals in my career, who always believed in me.

➤ In memory of Bill Smyth, a truly "extraordinary ordinary" man and one of the best guidance counselors and individuals I have ever known.

➤ Susan Kolwicz, my editor, who continues to make my life of writing books so easy through her organization, efficiency, helpful manner, and good humor.

Roger Pierangelo

➤ Marion Levine, Executive Director of North Shore Child and Family Guidance Center, who set me on the path into the world of special education.

➤ Renee Trachtenberg, Coordinator of Supported Work (Nassau BOCES) and her staff, who gave freely of their expertise in supported employment.

➤ Niomi Glaser, Coordinator of Special Education Training Resource Center Nassau BOCES, who fostered my work with parents of children with special needs.

➤ Ed Crane, for his technical knowledge that guided me through the world of the Internet.

Rochelle Crane

PROFESSIONAL ACKNOWLEDGMENTS

In the course of writing this book we have encountered many professionally outstanding sources. It has been our experience that these resources have contributed, and continue to contribute, enormous information, support, guidance, and education to parents, students, and professionals in the area of special education. While we have used many worthwhile sources and sites, we would like to take this opportunity to acknowledge the following: National Information Center for Children and Youth With Disabilities (NICHCY), HEATH Resource Center (National Clearinghouse on Postsecondary Education for Individuals With Disabilities) ERIC Clearinghouse, ARC (formerly the Association for Retarded Citizens), Children and Adults With Attention Deficit Disorders (CH.A.D.D.) 499 NW 70th Avenue, Suite 109, Plantation, FL 33317, the Council for Exceptional Children (CEC), and the National Transition Network and Parents Advocacy Coalition for Educational Rights (PACER).

ABOUT THE AUTHORS

Roger Pierangelo has over twenty-five years' experience as a regular classroom teacher, school psychologist in the Herricks Public School system in New Hyde Park, NY, administrator of special education programs, full professor in the graduate special education department at Long Island University, private practitioner in psychology, member of Committees on Special Education, evaluator for the N.Y. State Education Department, director of a private clinic, and consultant to numerous private and public schools, PTA, and SEPTA groups.

Dr. Pierangelo earned his B.S. from St. John's University, M.S. from Queens College, Professional Diploma from Queens College, and Ph.D. from Yeshiva University. Currently, he is working as a psychologist, both in the schools and in private practice; teaching at the college; and serving as director of a private clinic.

Dr. Pierangelo is a member of the American Psychological Association, N.Y. State Psychological Association, Nassau County Psychological Association, New York State Union of Teachers, and Phi Delta Kappa.

Dr. Pierangelo is the author of *A Survival Kit for the Special Education Teacher* (1994) and *The Special Education Teacher's Book of Lists* (1995), and coauthor of *Parent's Complete Special Education Guide* (1996)—all published by The Center for Applied Research in Education. He is also the author of *301 Ways to Be a Loving Parent*, published by Shapolsky Publishers of New York.

Rochelle Crane, C.S.W., is a psychiatric social worker who for fifteen years was on the staff of the North Shore Child and Family Guidance Center, a mental health agency on the North Shore of Long Island. From 1985 to 1990 Ms. Crane was the coordinator of its learning disability team. She is currently in private practice, treating adolescents and adults. In her capacity as a consultant to Board of Cooperative Educational Services, she leads workshops for parents of children with special needs. Ms. Crane also teaches in-service courses for teachers.

Ms. Crane has a master's degree in Social Work from Adelphi University. She is a member of the National Association of Social Workers and the OrthoPsychiatric Association.

ABOUT THIS RESOURCE

PURPOSE OF THE GUIDE

There are two common crises in the lives of children with disabilities, their families and those professionals who work with them. The first turning point is when the children enter the special education system and the second is when they leave it. This book is geared toward helping this population as they prepare to leave the world of special education. To make a successful transition from the context of secondary school to the next phase—either further schooling or work—educators, families, and others must prepare themselves about issues that have to be addressed well in advance. They must become knowledgeable about resources that are available at the local, state, and federal levels during the transition phase of special education.

There are global issues in the transition process—issues that are common to all; however, there are also a great variety of specific personal needs that depend upon the personality and interests, and the nature and severity of the disability of the individual.

Complete Guide to Special Education Transition Services has been developed to help individuals through the very difficult and confusing process of transitioning students from school to adulthood. The process of transition and the services that are available have only recently been developed and utilized by school districts. The federal and individual state laws governing this requirement are also new—and always changing. Schools and institutions must now provide transitional IEPs and services for these students and their families; however, many are unaware or uninformed about procedures, rights, school responsibilities, organizations, current laws, and available support services within the school, as well as community, city, state, and government agencies.

While many local school districts offer some pamphlets or short manuals on transition, they focus only on local responsibilities and services. The purpose of this guide is to provide teachers, administrators, parents, and students with an enormous reference source that will include procedures, laws, school responsibilities, organizations, forms, legal requirements, parents' responsibilities, state and government agencies, and anything else necessary to help ease them through this process.

A parent of a disabled student faces a very difficult task when it comes to trying to maneuver through all the red tape, options, and forms involved in the special education process. Nowhere is that procedure more intense and important than in the transition of a child to adulthood. Faced with a lack of information and responsibilities not encountered previously, a parent tends to become very anxious about what will occur when the child with disabilities leaves the safety of the local school. The transition process begins when the student with disabilities reaches 13 or 14 and continues through 21 if necessary. Parents must know what to do every step of the way. *Complete Guide to Special Education Transition Services* also addresses that need.

HELPFUL AND UNIQUE FEATURES

Complete Guide to Special Education Transition Services presents the most up-to-date information possible. It is a unique guide for several reasons:

➤ Developmental, step-by-step approach takes readers through a variety of topics and procedures necessary for a realistic awareness of issues faced during the transitional process.

➤ Written in an easy-to-read format, the book contains a wealth of tried-and-true suggestions drawing on the authors' extensive experience.

➤ The material is presented in such a way that it allows readers to utilize its content to help offer to the student with disabilities the most appropriate services available during the transition phase.

➤ The focus is on the more practical and commonly encountered issues, avoiding any material that may be obscure and meaningless.

➤ Useful information can be immediately applied to the variety of experiences faced by those who work and live with children who are disabled.

➤ Practical guidelines and checklists will help students who plan to go to college or on to community employment.

➤ Readers are given a thorough explanation of the most recent laws governing transitional services.

➤ An in-depth explanation of the school's responsibilities in the transition process is included.

➤ Complete and practical procedures are offered for parents to follow during the transitional phase.

➤ Legal concerns that must be addressed during the transition phase are carefully discussed.

➤ Organizations and community agencies that offer help in the transition process are explained.

➤ Step-by-step explanations are given of the responsibilities and requirements involved in the transitional IEP.

➤ End-of-chapter glossaries define terms used in selected chapters that may be unfamiliar to the reader.

➤ References at the end of each chapter list books and other sources of useful information. A complete listing of state and government agencies that offer support and guidance during the transitional process is provided in the Appendixes.

HOW TO USE THIS GUIDE

Teachers and parents of special education children will find *Complete Guide to Special Education Transition Services* invaluable. It will assist them through every phase required to successfully make the most appropriate decisions involving the transition of students from school to adulthood.

The information presented enables readers to feel more secure and aware regarding the sometimes overwhelming process of transition and "aging out."

This guide has been organized by issues rather than specific disabilities since many of the issues address the similar needs of various disabilities. Furthermore, *Complete Guide to Special Education Transition Services* covers issues under the responsibility of the school district, for example, transitional IEPs and vocational assessments—as well as others that are strictly within the province of the family, for example, social skills, sexual issues, wills, and so on.

Last, this guide assists parents, and professionals working with their children, in finding the appropriate channels for the children. We know from our experience that parents need a great deal of support and practical information to help them make the best decisions for their children. This guide helps everyone involved through the process with step-by-step directions that cover the areas of greatest concern in an easily understood manner.

Roger Pierangelo and Rochelle Crane

CONTENTS

——————————————— *Chapter 3* ———————————————

VOCATIONAL EDUCATION PLANNING   31

Chapter 4

LIVING ARRANGEMENTS   61

Chapter 10

POSTSECONDARY EDUCATIONAL OPTIONS   155

Chapter 11

ESTATE PLANNING FOR PARENTS   167

_____ *Chapter 12* _____

INSURANCE ISSUES FOR PARENTS 185

_____ *Chapter 13* _____

FINANCIAL CONCERNS 193

APPENDICES 199

CONTENTS

1

FUNDAMENTALS OF TRANSITION SERVICES

This chapter covers the following topics:

➤ Intent of transition services

➤ Brief history of transitional legislation

➤ Introduction of transition services

➤ Self-determination

➤ Importance of keeping records

The last two decades have witnessed significant changes for people with disabilities, in large part because of the disability rights movement, which in many ways paralleled the civil rights movement. People with disabilities used to be thought of as "the invisible minority." They were overlooked and "hidden away." They were embarrassments—treated as objects of pity and shame. Now these individuals are taking their place in an inclusive society. Individuals with disabilities are now a presence in all the media, commercial advertising, and many forms of public life. Changes in the laws, and progress and technology, have helped make these advances possible. Despite these gains, the barriers to acceptance remain society's myths, fears, and stereotypes about the disabled. Consequently, the efforts for change must be viewed as an ongoing process. The implementation of transition services is a significant component of this pathway to acceptance.

As most adults know from their own experience, the period known as adolescence is probably the most difficult and unsettling period of adjustment in one's development. It is a time filled with physical, emotional, and social upheavals. Until a child leaves secondary school, a parent experiences a sense of protective control over the child's life. This protective guidance normally involves educational, medical, financial, and social input to assist the child's growth. When the child leaves this setting, a parent undergoes a personal struggle in "letting go." There is always a certain amount of apprehension associated with the child's entrance into the adult world, as the greater responsibility for adjustment now falls on the child and the parent's role diminishes.

For the child with a disability, this developmental period can be fraught with even greater apprehension for a variety of reasons. Depending on the nature and severity of the disability, parents may play more of an ongoing role in their child's life even after he or she leaves secondary education. Historically, parents and the children have spent years actively involved in IEP development and meetings, transitional IEP development, and CSE meetings concerning educational and developmental welfare. Depending on the mental competence (the capability to make reasoned decisions) of the child with disabilities, some parents may have to continue to make vital decisions affecting all aspects of their children's lives; they need not shy away, thinking that they are being too overprotective if they are involved in the child's life after the child leaves school. On the other hand, the parents of children not affected by diminished mental competence should use all their energies to encourage the child's steps toward independence.

Since planning for the future of a student with disabilities can arouse fear of the unknown, a parent may tend to delay addressing these issues and instead focus only on the present. It is our belief, however, that working through these fears and thinking about the child's best future interest will ensure a meaningful outcome. Regardless of the nature and severity of a disability, parents will be exposed to a transitional process during the child's school years that will provide a foundation for the adult world. This transitional process will include many facets of planning for the future and should be fully understood by everyone concerned each step of the way. Planning for the future is an investment in a child's well-being and the purpose of this book is to help you understand all the aspects of this important time.

INTENT OF TRANSITION SERVICES

For many years educators have been concerned about the lack of success in adult life for students with disabilities. Research has shown that a large proportion of special education students did not go for further training and often did not receive postschool support and services. As these children "aged out" (at age 21 students were no longer eligible for a free and appropriate education including services and support) of the educational system, the families felt that they were being dropped into a void. While there were many services out in the community, parents were left to their own devices and would find out about such services and supports by chance. Parents and students were confronted with a complex array of service options and resources, each with unique roles, services, funding sources, forms, and eligibility requirements. The need for a collaborative, readily accessible system was obvious.

What seemed to be missing was the bridge between a student's school system and services for postsecondary school life. As a result, the concept of transitional services was developed to provide students who have special needs with a more structured path to adulthood.

BRIEF HISTORY OF TRANSITION LEGISLATION

The Education of the Handicapped Act, Public Law (P.L.) 94-142, was passed by Congress in 1975 and amended by P.L. 99-457 in 1986 to ensure that all children with disabilities would have a free, appropriate public education available to them that would meet their unique needs. It was again amended in 1990, and the name was changed to IDEA (Individuals With Disabilities Education Act). In the spring of 1997, Congress passed bills reauthorizing IDEA.

IDEA (P.L. 101-476,) defines "children with disabilities" as having any of the following types of disabilities: autism, deafness, deaf-blindness, hearing impairments (including deafness), mental retardation, multiple disabilities, orthopedic impairments, other health impairments, serious emotional disturbance, specific learning disabilities, speech or language impairments, traumatic brain injury, and visual impairments (including blindness). These terms are defined in the regulations for IDEA, as described below.

1. AUTISM

A developmental disability significantly affecting verbal and nonverbal communication and social interaction, generally evident before age three, that adversely affects educational performance.

2. DEAFNESS

A hearing impairment which is so severe that a child is impaired in processing linguistic information through hearing, with or without amplification, which adversely affects educational performance.

3. DEAF-BLINDNESS

Simultaneous hearing and visual impairments, the combination of which causes such severe communication and other developmental and educational problems that a child cannot be accommodated in special education programs solely for children with deafness or children with blindness.

4. HEARING IMPAIRMENT

A hearing impairment, whether permanent or fluctuating, which adversely affects a child's educational performance but which is not included under the definition of "deafness."

5. MENTAL DISABILITY

Significantly subaverage general intellectual functioning existing concurrently with deficits in adaptive behavior and manifested during the developmental period, which adversely affects a child's educational performance.

6. MULTIPLE DISABILITIES

Simultaneous impairments (such as mental retardation/blindness, mental retardation/orthopedic impairment, etc.), the combination of which causes such severe educational problems that the child cannot be accommodated in a special education program solely for one of the impairments. The term does not include children with deaf-blindness.

7. ORTHOPEDIC IMPAIRMENT

A severe orthopedic impairment which adversely affects a child's educational performance. The term includes impairments caused by a congenital anomaly (e.g., clubfoot, absence of some member, etc.), impairments caused by disease (e.g., poliomyelitis, bone tuberculosis, etc.), and impairments from other causes (e.g., cerebral palsy, amputations, and fractures or burns which cause contractures).

8. OTHER HEALTH IMPAIRMENT

Having limited strength, vitality or alertness, due to chronic or acute health problems such as a heart condition, tuberculosis, rheumatic fever, nephritis, asthma, sickle cell anemia, hemophilia, epilepsy, lead poisoning, leukemia, or diabetes, which adversely affects a child's educational performance. According to the Office of Special Education and

Rehabilitative Services' clarification statement of September 16, 1991, eligible children with ADD may also be classified under "other health impairment."

9. SERIOUS EMOTIONAL DISABILITY

(I.) A condition exhibiting one or more of the following characteristics over a long period of time and to a marked degree, which adversely affects educational performance (A) an inability to learn which cannot be explained by intellectual, sensory, or health factors; (B) an inability to build or maintain satisfactory interpersonal relationships with peers and teachers; (C) inappropriate types of behavior or feelings under normal circumstances; (D) a general pervasive mood of unhappiness or depression; or (E) a tendency to develop physical symptoms or fears associated with personal or school problems. (II.) The term includes children who have schizophrenia. The term does not include children who are socially maladjusted, unless it is determined that they have a serious emotional disturbance.

10. SPECIFIC LEARNING DISABILITY

A disorder in one or more of the basic psychological processes involved in understanding or in using language, spoken or written, which may manifest itself in an imperfect ability to listen, think, speak, read, write, spell, or do mathematical calculations. The term includes such conditions as perceptual disabilities, brain injury, minimal brain dysfunction, dyslexia, and developmental aphasia. The term does not include children who have learning problems which are primarily the result of visual, hearing, or motor disabilities, of mental retardation, of emotional disturbance, or of environmental, cultural, or economic disadvantage.

11. SPEECH OR LANGUAGE IMPAIRMENT

A communication disorder such as stuttering, impaired articulation, a language impairment, or a voice impairment, which adversely affects a child's educational performance.

12. TRAUMATIC BRAIN INJURY

An injury to the brain caused by an external physical force, resulting in total or partial functional disability or psychosocial maladjustment, or both, which adversely affects educational performance. The term does not include brain injuries that are congenital or degenerative, or brain injuries induced by birth trauma.

13. VISUAL IMPAIRMENT—INCLUDING BLINDNESS

A visual impairment which, even with correction, adversely affects a child's educational performance. The term includes both children with partial sight and those with blindness.

INTRODUCTION OF TRANSITION SERVICES

In 1992, the laws governing the education of children with disabilities took a major step forward with the introduction of transition services. The rules and regulations for IDEA released in 1992 define transition services as:

A.   A coordinated set of activities for a student, designed within an outcome-oriented process that promotes movement from school to postschool activities, including postsecondary education, vocational training, integrated employment (including supported employment), continuing and adult education, adult services, independent living, or community participation.

B. The coordinated set of activities must

➤ be based on the individual student's needs, taking into account the student's preferences and interests

➤ include instruction, community experience, the development of employment and other postschool adult living objectives and if appropriate, acquisition of daily living skills and functional evaluation. (IDEA PL101-476, 34 CFR 300.18)

Simply put, transition is

➤ helping students and family think about their life after high school and identify long-range goals

➤ designing the high school experience to ensure that students gain the skills and connections they need to achieve these goals

➤ the provision of funds and services to local school districts to assist in the transition process

In May 1994, President Clinton signed the School to Work Opportunities Act. This act has the blueprint to empower all individuals, including those with disabilities, to acquire the skills and experiences they need to compete. This landmark bill demonstrates that transition is clearly now a national priority, important to ensure our economic viability as well as offer *every* young person a chance at a productive life.

Every state receives federal special education moneys through Part B of IDEA, and in turn, most of these funds "flow through" to local school districts and other state-supported programs providing special education services. As a requirement of receiving these funds, state education agencies monitor the programs for which the funds are made available.

What Are Transition Services?

Transition services are aimed at providing students and their families with the practical and experiential skills and knowledge that will assist in a successful transition to adult life. While transition services are provided in each of the following areas, it is important to understand that not every student with disabilities will need to receive all of these services. The available services included in the transition process are:

➤ instruction

➤ employment

➤ postschool activities

➤ community experiences

and if appropriate:

➤ activities of daily living

➤ functional vocational evaluations

Some students with severe disabilities will need more extensive intervention for transition to adult life. Students with milder disabilities may require only limited services in only one or two of the above areas, with specific attention given to how the disability affects a particular aspect of transition.

Transition service regulations have to do with communication, collaboration, and coordination of plans, programs, services, supports, and resources. This communication, collaboration, and coordination must occur among students, families, schools, agencies, and communities. Together, they make decisions as well as share responsibilities and resources. All this is based on what is needed by and in the best interest of each student.

SELF-DETERMINATION: MAKING THEIR OWN CHOICES AND DECISIONS

One of the most significant concepts to emerge in the last few decades is the awareness of the importance of self-determination in the life of a disabled individual. For too long, decisions for disabled people were made by professionals with little input from the individual or parents. While these decisions were motivated by good intentions, they may have overlooked the desires, hopes, and aspirations that remained hidden within the person with disabilities. As our society has become more sensitive to the needs and rights of the disabled, we have moved to the concept of self-determination as a crucial element in the design of a life plan.

Self-determination is a person's ability to control his or her own destiny. A crucial part of the concept of self-determination involves the combination of attitudes and abilities that will lead children or individuals to set goals for themselves, and to take the initiative to reach these goals. To do this one must

➤ be in charge, which is not necessarily the same thing as self-sufficiency or independence

➤ make his or her own choices

➤ learn to solve problems effectively

➤ take control and responsibility for his or her life

➤ learn to experience and cope with the consequences of making decisions on his or her own

The Development of Self-Determination Skills

The development of self-determination skills is a process that begins in childhood and continues throughout one's life. It must be fully understood by parents when a child is still in school. This process begins early, so that the child learns how to grow up as a self-advocate and not be afraid to voice his or her needs, concerns, and opinions.

Parents of children with adequate mental competence sometimes "protect" them by making all their decisions. Parents interested in developing self-determination skills for their children must help them learn to

➤ set goals

➤ evaluate options

➤ make choices

➤ work to achieve goals

➤ practice self-determination experiences by offering opportunities for decision making, socialization, leisure activities, and more

➤ explore employment and housing options

➤ explore community recreation programs in their community by utilizing their own network of relatives and friends, as well as formal service systems

➤ take an active role in the decisions that will determine their future—even if it means allowing them to make mistakes.

Readers of this guide are urged to share the information found here with children with disabilities as they reach age-appropriate levels.

IMPORTANCE OF KEEPING RECORDS

It is extremely important that parents and students develop a recordkeeping system. This system should encompass three specific categories:

➤ Official documents

➤ Financial documents

➤ Chronicle of information

The first category, official documents, involves maintaining a file of a child's written official documents. Examples include

➤ all high school transcripts

➤ evaluations, tests

➤ medical records

➤ letters of recommendation

➤ job coach reports

➤ on-the-job training reports

➤ teacher comments

➤ schedules

➤ therapist reports

➤ IEPs

➤ transitional IEPs

➤ end-of-the-year reports

The second category, financial documents, includes

➤ sources of income and assets (pension funds, interest income, etc.)

➤ Social Security and Medicare information

- ➤   investment income

- ➤   insurance information with policy numbers

- ➤   bank accounts

- ➤   location of safe deposit boxes

- ➤   copies of recent income tax returns

- ➤   liabilities: what is owed to whom and when payments are due

- ➤   credit card and charge account names and numbers

- ➤   property taxes

- ➤   location of personal items

Refer to Chapters 11 through 13—Estate Planning, Insurance Issues, and Financial Concerns—for additional information on this important subject.

The third category involves an ongoing chronicle of information gathered as the result of

- ➤   phone conversations with school or agency officials

- ➤   summary of meetings

- ➤   copies of letters written by parents

- ➤   copies of letters received

- ➤   brochures handed out by organizations

A FINAL WORD

The chapters that follow alert parents, students, and professionals to the variety of important issues that they will face in the coming years. During this process, it is important to remain proactive, informed, involved, and hopeful.

When what you need doesn't exist, form bonds and join groups with others in the same situation. It has only been through personal struggles and efforts of parents, professionals, and individuals with disabilities that laws and attitudes have changed.

Initially, the collaborative efforts of parents and professionals best meet the needs of young children with disabilities. As these children enter the adult world, however, they should become partners in this collaborative team to promote their own well-being.

— GLOSSARY —

advocate—a person who pleads another's cause, a person who speaks or writes in support of something.

collaboration—working cooperatively with others to achieve common goals.

congenital anomaly—a condition existing at or before birth, resulting in a deviation or departure from the normal.

contracture—an abnormal, often permanent shortening—as of muscle—that results in deformity, especially in a joint of the body.

developmental aphasia—partial or total loss of the ability to articulate ideas or comprehend written or spoken language, present from birth as opposed to resulting from an injury or accident.

developmental disability—a severe chronic physical or mental incapacity such as cerebral palsy, arising before adulthood and usually lasting throughout life.

dyslexia—a learning disorder marked by impairment of the ability to recognize written words.

linguistics—of or relating to language.

outcome-oriented process—begins with the outcome statement and has a life span that exceeds the one-year life of the IEP. The outcome statement is *NOT* a behavioral objective or a goal statement; it is a destination statement pointing to where that student will be several years in the future. As the student approaches graduation, this statement will be refined and made more specific. All outcome statements are based on the student's preferences, interests, and needs.

supported employment—employment in which your child will need long-term or ongoing help to keep a job. (Refer to Chapter 3, Vocational Education Planning, for a complete explanation.)

— GENERAL REFERENCES —

"General Information About Disabilities Which Qualify Children and Youth for Special Education Services Under the IDEA Act." *News Digest 1995*. National Information Center for Children and Youth With Disabilities (NICHCY), P.O. Box 1492, Washington, DC 20013, (800)695-0285.

Introduction to Youth With Disabilities: Bibliography for Professionals, Feb. 1990. National Center for Youth With Disabilities, Publications, University of Minnesota, Box 721, 420 Delaware Street SE, Minneapolis, MN 55455, (612)626-2825.

The Network News Summer 1996. National Transition Network, Institute on Community Integration, University of Minnesota, Minneapolis, MN, 55455, (612)626-8200.

Nisbet, Jan. 1991. *Natural Supports in School, at Work, and in the Community for People With Severe Disabilities*. Paul H. Brookes, Baltimore. Code: Resources for Families.

O'Connell, Mary. 1992. *Getting Connected: How to Find Out About Groups and Organizations in Your Neighborhoods*. Center for Urban Affairs and Policy Research, Northwestern University, 2040 Sheridan Road, Evanston, IL 60208-4100. Topic Code: Community Integration.

The Pocket Guide to Federal Help: For Individuals With Disabilities. 1993. Clearinghouse on Disability Information, Office of Special Education and Rehabilitative Services, U.S. Department of Education, Room 3132 Switzer Building, Washington, DC 20202-2524.

"Questions and Answers About IDEA." *News Digest 1991*. National Information Center for Children and Youth With Disabilities (NICHCY), P.O. Box 1492, Washington, DC 20013, (800)695-0285.

Self-Advocacy Groups: 1994-95 Directory for North America. 1994. This publication lists the addresses and phone numbers of over 700 self-advocacy groups and organizations in the United States, Canada, and Mexico. Edited by Mary F. Hayden and Dick Senese. Available from

Publications Office, Institute on Community Integration, University of Minnesota, 150 Pillsbury Drive SE, Minneapolis, MN 55455, (612)624-4512.

Shapiro, J. 1993. *No Pity: People With Disabilities Forging a New Civil Rights Movement.* New York: Random House.

— REFERENCES ON LEGISLATION —

Carl D. Perkins Vocational Education Act, 20 U.S.C. Sections 2331-2342.

Code of Federal Regulations (C.F. R.): Title 34, Education, Parts 1 to 499, July 1986. Washington, DC: U.S. Government Printing Office.

Developmental Disabilities Assistance and Bill of Rights Act, 42 U.S.C. Section 6012.

Education of the Handicapped Act, 20 U.S.C. Sections 1400-1485.

Office of Special Education and Rehabilitative Services. Summary of existing legislation affecting persons with disabilities. Washington, DC: Clearinghouse on Disability Information. (An updated edition of this book is available from the Clearinghouse on Disability Information, Office of Special Education and Rehabilitative Services, 330 C Street, SW, Room 3132, Switzer Bldg., Washington, DC 20202-2319.)

Public Law 94-142 Education of the Handicapped Act, 1975.

Public Law 99-372, Handicapped Children's Protection Act of 1986.

Public Law 101-476, Individuals With Disabilities Education Act, 1990.

Public Law 100-407, Technology-Related Assistance for Individuals With Disabilities Act of 1988.

Public Law 101-127, Children With Disabilities Temporary Care Reauthorization Act of 1989.

Public Law 101-336, Americans With Disabilities Act of 1990.

Rehabilitation Act of 1973, 29 U.S.C. Sections 504, 701-794.

U.S. Department of Education. 1995. *Seventeenth Annual Report to Congress on the Implementation of the Individuals With Disabilities Education Act.* Washington, DC (Available from the Superintendent of Documents, U.S. Government Printing Office, Washington, DC 20402.)

— SELF-DETERMINATION REFERENCES —

Become Your Own Expert! Self-Advocacy Curriculum for Individuals With Learning Disabilities. 1995. Winnelle D. Carpenter, ed. Available from Minnesota Education Services, 70 County Road B2 West, Little Canada, MN 55117, (612)483-4442.

Choices: A Parent's View, Choices: A Consumer's View. 1992. Marge Goldberg and LeAnn Dahl. Available from PACER Center, 4826 Chicago Ave. S., Minneapolis, MN 55417, (612)827-2966.

"A Conceptual Framework for Enhancing Self-Determination." 1994. B. Abery. In *Challenges for a Service System in Transition: Ensuring Quality Community Experiences for Persons With Developmental Disabilities.* M. Hayden and B. Abery, eds. Paul H. Brookes, Baltimore, (800)638-3775.

A Curriculum Guide for the Development of Self-Determination and Advocacy Skills. 1994. Debora Ahern-Preslieu and Lisa Glidden. Available from A. J. Pappanikou Center, 62 Washington Street, Middletown, CT 06457, (860)344-7500.

A Guide to Enhancing the Self-Determination of Transition-Age Youth With Disabilities. 1994. B. Abery, A. Eggebeen, E. Rudrud, K. Arndt, and L. Tetu. Institute of Community Integration, University of Minnesota, 109 Pattee Hall, 150 Pillsbury Dr. SE, Minneapolis, MN 55455, (612)624-4512.

IMPACT: Feature Issue on Self-Advocacy. 1994. Publications Office, Institute on Community Integration, University of Minnesota, 150 Pillsbury Drive SE, Minneapolis, MN 55455, (612)624-4512.

IMPACT: Feature Issue on Self-Determination. 1993/94. Publications Office, Institute on Community Integration, University of Minnesota, 150 Pillsbury Drive SE, Minneapolis, MN 55455, (612)624-4512.

In Their Own Words. 1993. Produced by the Council on Education. Available from HEATH Resource Center, One Dupont Circle, Washington, DC 10036-1193, (800)544-3284.

Living Your Own Life. 1994. PACER, 4826 Chicago Ave. S., Minneapolis, MN 55417, (612)827-2966.

Self-Advocacy: Four Easy Pieces. 1993. Advocating Change Together, 1821 University Ave., #S-363, St. Paul, MN 55104, (612)641-0297.

"Self-Determination and the Education of Students With Mental Retardation." 1992. M. Wehmeyer. In *Education and Training in Mental Retardation,* 27, pp. 302-314.

"Self-Determination Revisited: Going Beyond Expectations." 1991. M. Ward. In *Transition Summary,* 7, National Information Center for Handicapped Children and Youth, Washington, DC, pp. 3-5, 12.

Taking Charge: Teenagers Talk About Life and Physical Disabilities. 1992. Woodbine House, 5625 Fishers Lane, Rockville, MD 20852, (800)843-7323.

WE CAN DO IT! A Curriculum for Teaching Self-Determination. Produced by Wilderness Inquiry and the Institute on Community Integration for the Minnesota Department of Education in November 1994. Available from Minnesota Education Services at Capitol View Center, 70 West Co. Rd. B2, Little Canada, MN 55117-1402, (612)483-4442.

Yes I Can Program. 1994. Institute on Community Integration, University of Minnesota, Publications Office, 109 Pattee Hall, 150 Pillsbury Drive SE, Minneapolis, MN 55455, (612)624-4512.

2

TRANSITIONAL IEPS—PLANS TO HELP STUDENTS' TRANSITION FROM SCHOOL TO ADULT LIFE

In this chapter you will learn about:

➤ When transition services must be provided

➤ Who determines what services are needed

➤ Where the transitional process takes place

➤ Individualized transitional education program (ITEP)

➤ Adult service providers

➤ The role of the family in the transition process

➤ Transition planning time line

➤ Transition checklist

➤ Sample transitional individual education plan

➤ Commonly asked questions and answers about transition services

WHEN TRANSITION SERVICES MUST BE PROVIDED

While the specific start date may vary from state to state and district to district, the federal guidelines state that schools *must* begin to provide transition services no later than age 16. A school may provide transition services to younger students, however, when their needs deem it appropriate. This may be particularly important for students with severe disabilities, or for those who are at risk of dropping out of school at or prior to age 16. The transition process may begin at the junior high school or middle school level. This process culminates with a high school diploma, IEP diploma, or certificate of attendance.

WHO DETERMINES WHAT SERVICES ARE NEEDED

The regulations of IDEA are very clear as to which individuals should participate in determining the transition services a student needs and what these services will entail. The following participants are usually present at the transition IEP meeting:

- the student's classroom teacher
- a school representative
- the parent(s)
- the student
- participating agencies

This chapter will help you understand the requirements for Transitional IEPs under the Individuals With Disabilities Education Act (IDEA). It was also developed to acquaint readers with each of the sections within the law and the proposed rules and regulations that directly relate to transition. This chapter tells you how the transitional IEP is an integral part of a child's transition process; its purpose is to summarize the key components of transition services and to assist with planning and implementing a child's transitional services.

WHERE THE TRANSITIONAL PROCESS TAKE PLACE

The transitional IEP process follows a child through middle school and high school. It usually takes place at the annual review meeting of the CSE. During this meeting, the transitional IEP coordinator will be present and assist the family in determining the appropriate services and experiences for a child at that particular stage and at future stages.

Districts are required to develop and implement a strategic plan for incorporating transition services within the individualized education program (IEP) process. The Committee on Special Education (CSE) must identify postschool outcomes for a child and include activities in the transitional IEP that prepare for the child's participation in the adult community.

INDIVIDUALIZED TRANSITIONAL EDUCATION PROGRAM (ITEP)

The IEP, as it has been defined over the years by legislation and court rulings, is not changed by the presence of the transition services section. The IEP is still a contract between the students, the parents, and the school. It is not a performance contract; the IEP spells out what the school will do (services and activities). If it is written on the IEP, the school is responsible for performing this stated service activity.

The IEP should carry only the information about transition services that the school district can provide, directly or indirectly (by arranging for another agency to provide services coordinated with the school services).

As in previous interpretations of the IEP, parents cannot be listed as responsible for achieving an outcome or providing a service. The school district is responsible for this.

The ITEP is a part of the overall IEP but represents a very important piece in determining a child's future. The ITEP should include long-term adult outcomes from which annual goals and objectives are defined.

The following should be addressed in the ITEP:

1. A statement of transition services should be responsive to your child's preferences, interests, and needs. The beginning date for the service should be included.

2.　Annual goals and objectives could include the following ten areas:

- legal/advocacy—guardianship
- independence/residential—private residence vs. group home
- recreation/leisure—joining sports activities
- financial/income—banking and checking accounts
- medical/health—health insurance, physician selection
- employment—sheltered workshop vs. competitive employment
- transportation—public vs. private
- postsecondary/continuing education—college vs. vocational training
- other support needs—clergy, fraternal organizations

3.　Long-term adult outcomes in the IEP should include statements on the child regarding his or her performance in employment, postsecondary education, and community living.

4.　A coordinated set of activities must be included in the ITEP. They must demonstrate the use of various strategies, including community experiences and adult living objectives. If one of these activities is not included in the IEP in a particular year, then the IEP must explain why that activity is not reflected in any part of the student's program. Activities of daily living and functional vocational evaluation activities should also be included.

5.　A list of participants involved in the planning and development of the Individualized Transitional Educational Program should be made available to all participants.

ADULT SERVICE PROVIDERS

Adult service providers encompass a wide range of programs and agencies. These are comprehensive nonprofit agencies providing residential, employment, and recreational opportunities that vary from state to state, and from community to community. They may be the recipients of government funds, supplemented by nongovernment sources (e.g., client fees, insurance payments, United Way allocations, or donations). These agencies also vary as to the range of programs they offer. Some providers service only people with specific disabilities, while others cover many disabilities.

Further information on these adult service providers can be found in the Appendixes.

THE ROLE OF THE FAMILY IN THE TRANSITION PROCESS

Listed below are steps that a family can take to assist in the transitional process:

➤　Explore your community for useful community resources.

➤　Discuss transition options with other families who have been through this process.

➤　Seek out information about occupational, educational, and living options.

➤　Work with the school in finding ways to increase your child's academic, career, and personal independence skills.

➤ Set achievable goals for your child.

➤ Help your child develop the ability to communicate his or her needs, preferences, and interests to school staff and other professionals.

➤ Observe the kinds of things your child can do independently and the areas in which he or she may need assistance.

➤ Participate actively in meetings with the school and other professionals.

➤ Make sure you plan and prepare well in advance for your child's future financial, medical, and housing resource needs, as appropriate by: (a) assisting with application for Social Security Disability or Supplemental Security Income (SSI) benefits; (b) developing a will; (c) determining guardianship; (d) applying for financial aid for postsecondary education or training. (All of these issues are discussed in detail in further chapters.)

➤ Help your child obtain key identification documents—a social security card, driver's license, or nondriver identification card.

➤ Help your child develop independent decision-making and communication skills.

➤ Help your child explore options and set realistic goals for the future.

➤ Enhance your child's positive self-esteem and assist him or her in developing independence, including self-reliance, self-advocacy, and self-management skills.

➤ Use actual home-life opportunities to teach your child daily living skills, for example, banking, shopping, cooking, cleaning, laundry.

➤ Promote good money management, budgeting, and savings.

➤ Encourage your child to become aware of the world of work.

➤ Help your child to locate and obtain a part-time job.

➤ Reinforce work-related behaviors at home (grooming, etiquette, following directions, completing chores, etc.).

➤ Provide opportunities for such leisure time activities as sports, daily exercise, or hobbies.

➤ Encourage your child to participate in social activities with peers.

➤ Teach your child how to utilize community-based resources (library, recreation, transportation, stores, etc.).

➤ Work actively with your CSE to make sure the plan is successful.

➤ Stay in close contact with your child's teachers.

TRANSITION PLANNING TIME LINE

The following series of events must be considered during a child's transition process. All items will not be applicable to all students or to all state regulations. The list is provided to serve as an optional planning tool.

Transition Planning Time Line

AGE RANGE	ACTION

12–15

_____ Initiate vocational assessment.

_____ Develop and implement strategies to increase responsibilities and independence at home.

_____ Discuss the following curriculum areas at CSE meetings:

        Academic

        Social

        Language/communication

        Occupational

        Self-help skills

        Self-advocacy skills

14–16

_____ Introduce and discuss transition services.

_____ Notify parents that transition services will be incorporated into the IEP, beginning at age 15.

_____ Assure that copies of work-related documents are available:

        Social security card

        Birth certificate

        Working papers (if appropriate)

_____ Obtain parental consent so that the appropriate adult agency representative can be involved.

_____ Develop transition component of IEP, and annually thereafter.

_____ Complete periodic vocational evaluations.

15–21

_____ Discuss adult transition with CSE.

_____ Consider summer employment or volunteer experience.

_____ Explore community leisure activities.

_____ Consider the need for residential opportunities, including completing applications, as appropriate.

_____ Complete periodic vocational evaluations.

16–21

_____ Obtain personal ID card.

_____ Obtain driver's training and license.

AGE RANGE		ACTION

16–21 *(cont'd)*   _____   Develop transportation/mobility.
strategies such as:

> Independent travel skills training
> Public or paratransit transportation
> Needs for travel attendant

_____   Investigate SSDI/SSI/Medicaid programs.

_____   Consider guardianship or emancipation.

_____   Develop and update employment plans.

_____   Involve state vocational rehabilitation agencies, as appropriate within two years of school exit.

_____   Research possible adult living situations.

_____   Investigate postschool opportunities (further educational vocational training, college, military, etc.)

_____   Complete periodic vocational evaluations.

18–21   _____   Seek legal guardianship.

_____   Apply for postschool college and other training programs.

_____   Male students register for the draft (no exceptions).

_____   Register to vote.

_____   Review health insurance coverage: inform insurance company of child's disability and investigate rider of continued eligibility.

_____   Complete transition to employment, further education or training, and community living, affirming that arrangements are in place for the following:

> Postsecondary/continuing education
> Employment
> Legal/advocacy
> Personal independence/residential
> Recreation/leisure
> Medical/health
> Counseling
> Financial/income
> Transportation/independent travel skills
> Other

© 1997 by The Center for Applied Research in Education

TRANSITION CHECKLIST

Families may wish to consider the following checklist of transition activities when preparing transition plans with the IEP team. The student's skills and interests will determine which items on the checklist are relevant and whether these transition issues should be addressed at IEP transition meetings. The checklist can also help identify who should be part of the IEP transition team. Responsibility for carrying out the specific transition activities should be determined at the IEP transition meetings.

Four to Five Years Before Leaving the School District

➢ Identify personal learning styles and the necessary accommodations if the child is to be a successful learner and worker.

➢ Identify career interests and skills, complete interest and career inventories, and identify additional education or training requirements.

➢ Explore options for postsecondary education and admission criteria.

➢ Identify interests and options for future living arrangements, including supports.

➢ Learn to help the child communicate his or her interests, preferences, and needs effectively.

➢ Teach the student how to explain his or her disability and the necessary accommodations.

➢ Learn and practice informed decision-making skills.

➢ Investigate assistive technology tools that can increase community involvement and employment opportunities.

➢ Broaden the child's experiences with community activities and help him or her form friendships.

➢ Pursue and use transportation options.

➢ Investigate money management and identify necessary skills.

➢ Acquire identification card and the ability to communicate personal information.

➢ Identify and begin learning skills necessary for independent living.

➢ Learn and practice personal health care.

Two to Three Years Before Leaving the School District

➢ Identify community support services and programs (vocational rehabilitation, county services, centers for independent living, etc.).

➢ Invite adult service providers, peers, and others to the IEP transition meeting.

➢ Match career interests and skills with vocational course work and community work experiences.

➢ Gather more information on postsecondary programs and the support services offered, and make arrangements for accommodations to take college entrance exams.

➢ Identify health care providers and become informed about sexuality and family planning issues.

➢ Determine the need for financial support (Supplemental Security Income, state financial supplemental programs, Medicare).

➢ Learn and practice appropriate interpersonal, communication, and social skills for different settings (employment, school, recreation, with peers, etc.).

➢ Explore legal status with regard to decision making prior to age of majority—wills, guardianship, special needs trust.

➢ Begin a résumé and update it as needed.

➢ Practice independent living skills—budgeting, shopping, cooking, and housekeeping.

➢ Identify needed personal assistant services, and if appropriate, learn to direct and manage these services.

One Year Before Leaving the School District (for the Child)

➢ Apply for financial support programs. (Supplemental Security Income, vocational rehabilitation, and personal assistant services).

➢ Identify the postsecondary school plan and arrange for accommodations.

➢ Practice effective communication by developing interview skills, asking for help, and identifying necessary accommodations at postsecondary and work environments.

➢ Specify desired job and obtain paid employment with supports as needed.

➢ Take responsibility for arriving on time to work, appointments, and social activities.

➢ Assume responsibility for health care needs (making appointments, filling and taking prescriptions, etc.).

➢ Register to vote (and for selective service if a male).

SAMPLE TRANSITIONAL IEP

STUDENT TRANSITION ACTION PLAN—PAGE 1

Descriptive Information: _____ Date Plan Initiated: _____

Student Name: _____ Age: _____ DOB: _____

Case Coordinator: _____

Social Security #: _____ Disability: _____

Phone: _____

Parent/guardian name: _____ Mother's/Father's home phone #: _____

Home address: _____ Mother's/Father's work phone #: _____

Grade: _____ Teacher: _____ County of residence: _____

Class location: _____ School phone: _____ Social worker: _____

Vocational education placement: _____ Home school district: _____

Contact person (name and phone): _____ Contact person (CSE): _____

Additional vocational/technical placements/program: _____

_____

_____

Additional Services Needed: _____

_____

_____

PARTICIPANTS in TRANSITION PLANNING

Name	Role/Agency
_____	_____
_____	_____
_____	_____

Employment Responsibilites	*Date*	*Activities Accomplished*
____ Competitive Employment (no need for services)	_____	_____
____ Competitive Employment (time-limited support)	_____	_____
____ Supported Employment (infrequent support)	_____	_____
____ Supportive Employment (daily support)	_____	_____
____ Sheltered Workshop	_____	_____
____ Day Treatment	_____	_____
____ Volunteer Work	_____	_____
____ Summer Employment	_____	_____
____ Other	_____	_____
____ Not Applicable	_____	_____

Postsecondary Education and Training

____ Community College or University (no support needed)	_____	_____
____ Community College or University (support needed)	_____	_____
____ Technical/Trade School (no support needed)	_____	_____
____ Technical /Trade School (support needed)	_____	_____
____ Adult Education Classes	_____	_____
____ Other	_____	_____
____ Not Applicable	_____	_____

Residential

____ Parents or Relatives	_____	_____
____ Intermediate Care Facility	_____	_____
____ Community Residence	_____	_____
____ Supervised Apartment	_____	_____
____ Supported Apartment	_____	_____
____ Independent Living	_____	_____
____ Foster Care/Family Care	_____	_____
____ Respite	_____	_____
____ Section 8 Housing	_____	_____
____ Other	_____	_____

STUDENT TRANSITION ACTION PLAN—PAGE 3

Transportation	Date	Activities Completed	Responsibilities
___ Independent			
___ Family Transportation			
___ Car Pool			
___ Public Transportation			
___ Specialized Transportation			
___ Agency Transportation			
___ Other			
___ Not Applicable			

Recreation/Leisure

___ Independent Recreation			
___ Family Supported Recreation			
___ Church Groups			
___ Local Clubs			
___ Community Parks and Recreation			
___ Specialized Recreation for Individuals With Disabilities			
___ Other			
___ Not Applicable			

Personal/Home/Money Management

___ Independent (no support needed)			
___ Citizenship Skills			
___ Insurance Coverage			
___ Money Management			
___ Use of Community Resources			
___ Meal Preparation			
___ Housekeeping Skills			
___ Self-Care			
___ Other			

Advocacy/Legal

___ Guardianship			
___ Wills/Trusts			
___ Self-Advocacy			
___ Client Assistance Program (CAP)			
___ Other			

23

Medical Responsibilities	*Date*	*Activities Completed*
____ Medical Care, Daily Care	_____	_____
____ Intermediate Care	_____	_____
____ Medical Services: General Check-ups, Specialists, Medical Supervision	_____	_____
____ Dental Care	_____	_____
____ Use of Free Clinics	_____	_____
____ Therapy (OT/PT. Sp./Lan.)	_____	_____
____ Family Insurance	_____	_____
____ Individual Insurance	_____	_____
____ Medicaid	_____	_____
____ Visiting Nurse/Home Health	_____	_____
____ Aide	_____	_____
____ Medication	_____	_____
____ Other	_____	_____

Social/Sexual

____ Individual Counseling	_____	_____
____ Group Counseling/Support	_____	_____
____ Family Planning Services	_____	_____
____ Other	_____	_____

Financial/Income

____ Earned Wages	_____	_____
____ Unearned Income (family support, gifts)	_____	_____
____ SSI/SSDI	_____	_____
____ Food Stamps, Housing Subsidy	_____	_____
____ Other	_____	_____

Communication

____ Braille	_____	_____
____ Assistive Technology	_____	_____
____ Computer Applications	_____	_____
____ Interpreter Services	_____	_____
____ Other	_____	_____

COMMONLY ASKED QUESTIONS AND ANSWERS
ABOUT TRANSITION SERVICES

1. **What are examples of postschool activities?**

   The term *postschool activities* describes what the student wants to do after high school: namely, where the student wants to live, work, recreate, and participate in his or her community.

2. **What are the requirements regarding consideration of the student's "preferences and interests" when developing the transition services for the IEP? How are the student's preferences and interests determined?**

   The student must have the opportunity to indicate his or her preferences and interests during the IEP meeting when transition services are being considered. If the student doesn't attend the IEP meeting when transition services are discussed, the district must ensure that the student's interests and preferences are considered during the development of the statement of needed transition services. To accomplish this, the school district may use checklists and other relevant self-assessments, including personal interviews and situational assessments. Family members and peers could also provide information to assist in determining a student's preferences and interests.

3. **Must each activity area be addressed at each annual review?**

   Yes. Instruction, community experiences, employment and other postschool adult living objectives, and, if appropriate, daily living skills and functional vocational evaluation must be addressed at each annual review.

4. **What are the school district's responsibilities for inviting students to IEP meetings that address transition services?**

   School districts are responsible for inviting students to their own IEP meetings. The invitation may be included in the parents' notification of the IEP meeting or it may be separate. Documentation of the student's invitation should be maintained in the student's record.

5. **Are there any circumstances under which a student would not be invited?**

   No. The rule clearly states that if a purpose of the meeting is to consider transition services for a student, the school district shall invite the student to attend the IEP meeting.

6. **Which agencies should be invited to the first IEP meeting?**

   School district personnel will have to rely on their best professional judgment and knowledge of adult agencies to determine which agencies to invite to the first meeting in which transition services are addressed. Copies of correspondence with invited agencies should be included in the student's records to document the invitation.

7. **What are participating agencies?**

   Relevant agencies could include vocational rehabilitation centers, developmental disabilities and regional providers, Job Training Partnership Act providers, community colleges, colleges and universities, and any other agency determined appropriate to provide transition services for a student with a disability.

8. *May IEP meetings concerning transition services be conducted if parents are not in attendance?*

   Yes. The IEP meeting may be conducted without the parent(s) in attendance if the school district is unable to obtain the attendance of the parents. The school district must have a record of its attempts to arrange a mutually agreed-upon time and place. If the parents cannot attend, steps shall be taken to ensure parent participation. Parent input on the IEP, including transition services, may be provided through face-to-face or telephone conferences, written correspondence, or other preplanning activities.

9. **What should the final IEP contain for a student with a disability?**

   The last IEP developed before the student is expected to leave school must contain the goals and objectives that are appropriate for the one-year period of time during which the IEP is in effect. All needed interagency responsibilities or linkages should be included.

10. **Once a student is no longer the responsibility of the school, who is responsible for providing transition services?**

    Designation of other participating agencies' responsibilities or linkages, or both, for providing services should be clearly stated in the IEP before the student leaves the school setting.

11. **Should needed transition services be identified when the services cannot be provided or are not available?**

    Yes. Needed transition services must be identified on the IEP based on the individual student's needs, preferences, and interests. The IEP committee should identify a student's transition strengths and needs regardless of known or unknown service providers. The team should brainstorm for strategies to meet the identified needs.

12. **Do the transition requirements extend to students protected under Section 504, but not served under IDEA?**

    No. Students protected under Section 504 are not required to have an IEP; however, students who previously were 504 eligible may now qualify under IDEA. If they need specially designed instruction in transition services, they may qualify for IDEA and have only transition services on the IEP.

13. **How do you resolve differences between parent and student on postschool outcomes?**

    Ultimately, the student's life goals are the ones being developed, and those should be given greater weight in the planning process. Attempts should be made, however, to achieve consensus through exploratory experiences and further discussions.

14. **Who decides what is actually written in the statement section on transition services? Who has the final decision?**

    The student, family, school, and appropriate agencies must decide together what the content will be. A successful transition depends on all parties' working cooperatively to develop and implement the programs, services, and activities in the ITEP.

A FINAL WORD

Transition services now provide individuals with disabilities the opportunities to choose goals, objectives, and activities that create a pathway to the future. The plan for this future lies in the structure of the transitional individual education plan. This plan has improved, and will continue to improve, the chances of success for individuals with disabilities, and further ensures their inclusion in the general population.

— GLOSSARY —

annual review meeting—a required yearly meeting of the Committee on Special Education to review the classification, program, and placement of a student with disabilities.

centers for independent living—organizations whose purpose is to promote and provide services to help persons with disabilities lead independent lives.

client—a person using the services of an agency. The more current term is "consumer."

Committee on special education—A state-mandated district committee whose responsibilities include overseeing programs and services for children with disabilities.

functional—tasks and activities relevant to daily life.

habilitation—the process of providing specific learning experiences for individuals with disabilities.

learning styles—the personal, environmental, and learning characteristics that enhance an individual's ability to learn, for example, structured vs. unstructured, perseverance, visual learner.

personal assistant services—agencies that provide service assistants to individuals with disabilities, for example, home health providers, readers.

Section 504—refers to Section 504 of the Rehabilitation Act of 1973 in which guarantees are provided for the civil rights of students and adults with disabilities. It also applies to the provision of services for children whose disabilities are not severe enough to warrant classification, but who could benefit from supportive services and classroom modifications—for example a physical or mental impairment substantially limiting one or more major life activity but not severe enough to warrant classification under IDEA (Individual Disability Education Act).

Social Security Disability Income—SSDI benefits are paid to persons who become disabled before the age of 22 if at least one of the parents had worked a certain amount of time under Social Security but is now disabled, retired, or deceased. The SSDI considers the employment status of the applicant's parents. As with SSI, eligibility for SSDI generally makes an individual eligible for food stamps and Medicaid benefits as well.

Social Security Insurance—the SSI program is a federally funded program targeted for individuals who are both (a) in financial need, and (b) blind or disabled. People who get SSI usually get food stamps and Medicaid, too.

vocational assessment—the techniques used to determine your child's interests, aptitudes, and skills.

vocational rehabilitation—a program designed to help disabled adults obtain and hold a job.

— REFERENCES —

Anderson, W.; Chitwood, S.; and Hayden, D. 1990. *Negotiating the Special Education Maze: A Guide for Parents and Teachers* (2d ed.). Rockville, MD: Woodbine House. [Available from Woodbine House, 6510 Bells Mill Road, Bethesda, MD 20817. Telephone: (800)843-7323; (301)897-3570.]

Black, J., and Ford, A. 1989. "Planning and Implementing Activity-Based Lessons." In A. Ford, R. Schnorr, L. Meyer, L. Davern, J. Black, and P. Dempsey (eds.), *The Syracuse Community-Referenced Curriculum Guide for Students With Moderate and Severe Disabilities* (pp. 295-311). Baltimore, MD: Paul H. Brookes.

Bullis, M., and Gaylord-Ross, R. 1991. *Moving on: Transitions for Youth With Behavioral Disorders.* Reston, VA: Council for Exceptional Children. [Available from the Council for Exceptional Children, 1920 Association Drive, Reston, VA 22091-1589. Telephone: (703)620-3660.]

Burke, Edward (ed.), National Council on Disability. 1995. *Improving the Implementation of the Individuals With Disabilities Education Act: Making Schools Work for All of America's Children.* Washington, DC: Author. [Available from National Council on Disability, 1331 F Street NW, Suite 1050, Washington, DC 20004-1107. Telephone: (202)272-2004.]

Copenhaver, J. 1995. *Section 504: An Educator's Primer: What Teachers and Administrators Need to Know About Implementing Accommodations for Eligible Individuals With Disabilities.* Logan, UT: Mountain Plains Regional Resource Center. [Available from the Mountain Plains RRC, 1780 North Research Parkway, Suite 112, Logan, UT 84341-9620. Telephone: (801)752-0238.]

Cutler, B. C. 1993. *You, Your Child, and "Special" Education: A Guide to Making the System Work.* Baltimore, MD: Paul H. Brookes. [Available from Paul H. Brookes Publishing Company, P.O. Box 10624, Baltimore, MD 21285-0624. Telephone: (800)638-3775.]

DeStefano, L., and Wermuth, T. R. 1992. "IDEA (P.L. 101-476): Defining a Second Generation of Transition Services." In F. R. Rusch, L. DeStefano, J. Chadsey-Rusch, L. A. Phelps, and E. Szymanshi (eds.), *Transition From School to Adult Life: Models, Linkages, and Policy* (pp. 537-549). Sycamore, IL: Sycamore Publishing. [Available from Sycamore Publishing Company, P.O. Box 133, Sycamore, IL 60178. Telephone: (815)756-5388.]

Elksnin, L., and Elksnin, N. 1990. "Using Collaborative Consultation With Parents to Promote Effective Vocational Programming." *Career Development for Exceptional Individuals,* 13(2), 135-142. [Available from the Division on Career Development, Council for Exceptional Children, 1920 Association Drive, Reston, VA 22091. Telephone: (703)620-3660.]

Falvey, M. A (ed.). 1989. *Community-Based Curriculum: Instructional Strategies for Students With Severe Handicaps* (2d ed.). Baltimore, MD: Paul H. Brookes.

Gould, M.; McTaggart, N.; and Rees, S. n.d. *Successful Transition From School to Work and Adult Life: A Handbook for Students, Parents, Teachers, and Advocates.* Baltimore: Self-advocacy Training Project of Maryland. [Available from Self-advocacy Training Project, Disabled in Action of Baltimore, 3000 Chestnut Avenue, Baltimore, MD 21211.]

Harnisch, D. L., and Fisher, A. T. (eds.). 1989. *Transition Literature Review: Educational, Employment, and Independent Living Outcomes.* Vol. 3. Champaign, IL: Secondary Transition Intervention Effectiveness Institute. [Available from Transition Research Institute at Illinois, University of Illinois at Urbana-Champaign, 61 Childrens Research Center, 51 Gerty Drive, Champaign, IL 61820. Telephone: (217)333-2325.]

Hartman, R. C. (ed.). 1991. "Transition in the United States: What's Happening." Information from *HEATH,* 10(3), 1, 4-6.

Johnson, B. H.; McGonigel, M. J.; and Kauffmann, R. K. 1991. *Guidelines and Recommended Practices for the Individualized Family Service Plan* (2d ed.). Bethesda, MD: Association for the Care of Children's Health. [Available from ACCH, 7910 Woodmont Avenue, Suite 300, Bethesda, MD 20814-3015. Telephone: (301)654-6549.]

Leach, L. N., and Harmon, A. 1990. *Annotated Bibliography on Transition From School to Work.* Vol. 5. Champaign, IL: Transition Research Institute. [Available from Transition Research Institute at Illinois, College of Education, University of Illinois at Urbana-Champaign, 61 Childrens Research Center, 51 Gerty Drive, Champaign, IL 61820. Telephone: (217)333-2325.]

McNair, J., and Rusch, F. R. 1991. "Parent Involvement in Transition Programs." *Mental Retardation,* 29(2), 93-101. [Available from the American Association on Mental Retardation, 1719 Kalorama Road NW, Washington, DC 20009. Telephone: (202)387-1968.]

National Easter Seal Society, East Lake Street, Chicago, IL 60601. Murphy, M. 1990. *Road Map to Transition for Young Adults With Severe Disabilities.* San Jose, CA: Santa Clara County Office of Education. (ERIC Document Reproduction Service No. ED 319 201.)

Nisbet, J. 1992. *Natural Supports in School, at Work, and in the Community for People With Severe Disabilities.* Baltimore, MD: Paul H. Brookes.

PACER Center. 1993. *Begin the Between: Planning for the Transition From High School to Adult Life.* PACER Center, 4825 Chicago Ave., South, Minneapolis, MN 55417. Topic: Resources for Families.

Repetto, J.; White, W.; and Snauwaert, D. 1990. "Individual Transition Plans (ITP): A National Perspective." *Career Education for Exceptional Individuals,* 13(2), 109-119.

Rusch, F. R.; Hughes, C.; and Kohler, P. D. 1991. *Descriptive Analysis of Secondary School Education and Transition Services Model Programs.* Champaign, IL: Secondary Transition Intervention Effectiveness Institute. [Available from Transition Research Institute at Illinois, University of Illinois at Urbana-Champaign, 61 Childrens Research Center, 51 Gerty Drive, Champaign, IL 61820. Telephone: (217)333-2325.]

Smith-Davis, J., and Littlejohn, W. R. 1991. "Related Services for School-Aged Children With Disabilities." *NICHCY News Digest,* 1(2). [Available from NICHCY.]

Trohanis, P. L. 1995. "Progress in Providing Services to Young Children With Special Needs and Their Families: An Overview to and Update on Implementing the Individuals With Disabilities Education Act." *NEC*TAS Notes,* Number 7, 1-20.

Wagner, M. March 1989. "The Transition Experiences of Youth With Disabilities: A Report From the National Longitudinal Transition Study." Paper presented at the annual meeting of the Council for Exceptional Children, San Francisco, CA. [Available from SRI International, 333 Ravenswood Avenue, Menlo Park, CA 94025. Telephone: (415)326-6200.]

Wandry, D., and Repetto, J. 1993. "Transition Services in the IEP." *NICHCY Transition Summary,* V(1), 1-28. [Available from NICHCY.]

Ward, M. J. 1992. "Introduction to Secondary Special Education and Transition Issues." In F. R. Rusch, L. DeStefano, J. Chadsey-Rusch, L. A. Phelps, and E. Szymanshi (eds.). *Transition From School to Adult Life: Models, Linkages, and Policy* (pp. 387-389). Sycamore, IL: Sycamore Publishing. [Available from Sycamore Publishing, P.O. Box 133, Sycamore, IL 60178. Telephone: (815)756-5388.]

Wehman, P. 1992. *Life Beyond the Classroom: Transition Strategies for Young People With Disabilities.* Baltimore, MD: Paul H. Brookes.

Wilson, N. O. 1992. *Optimizing Special Education: How Parents Can Make a Difference.* New York: Insight Books. [Available from Insight Books, Division of Plenum Press, 233 Spring Street, New York, NY 10013. Telephone: (800)221-9369.]

Young Adult Institute. n.d. *Parents as Transitional Specialists.* New York: Author. [Available from the Young Adult Institute, 460 W. 34th Street, New York, NY 10001. Telephone: (212)563-7474.]

3

VOCATIONAL EDUCATION PLANNING

This chapter covers the following topics:

➤ The specific professionals who are trained to help students with disabilities plan and prepare for employment

➤ Prevocational skills

➤ Training options such as internships and apprenticeships

➤ Vocational education plans

➤ Job coaches

➤ Assessing skills for possible employment

➤ The Division of Rehabilitation Services (DRS)

➤ What happens when parents contact a DRS agency

➤ Services provided by the DRS agency

➤ Rights and responsibilities with a DRS agency

➤ Resolving disagreements with a DRS agency

➤ Assessment options

➤ Level I, Level II, and Level III vocational assessments

➤ Supported employment

➤ Signals that may indicate a child's need for supported employment

➤ How social service agencies can help in the employment process

➤ Services provided by social service agencies

➤ The questions parents must ask the agency that helps their child find employment

➤ Situational assessments

➤ Functional assessments

➤ Vocational terms

➤ Laws protecting the employment rights of the disabled

Crossing the threshold from the world of school to the world of work brings a significant change in everyone's life. School is an entitlement, meaning that it is an environment that our system of government supplies for all of our citizens. The workplace is the opposite; no one is entitled to a job. The workplace is governed by the competitive market and students—whether disabled or not—have to be able to function in that setting, or they will not survive.

One of the most important aspects of transition planning is the preparation of students for the world of work. Up to now, the focus has been on helping him or her fulfill the educational requirements for graduation from a secondary school. Now comes a very real and practical issue that can create many concerns. With the proper information and resources this next phase of the transition process can also be rewarding. A parent must fully understand the options in order to help the child make the best decision for his or her future.

The purpose of this chapter is to familiarize readers with laws, procedures, resources, terminology, and other information that can assist you through this phase. We will help you identify types of services and programs, and sources of available support. We will also help you learn how to evaluate these options to determine the best for a child and his or her particular needs.

VOCATIONAL ASSESSMENTS

One of the techniques used to determine a child's interests, aptitudes, and skills is a vocational assessment. A vocational assessment is the responsibility of your district's special education program. It begins by assessing referrals for special education services and continues throughout subsequent annual reviews. The planning of transitional services includes the CSE's development of transitional employment goals and objectives based on the child's needs, preferences, and interests. These will be identified through the child-centered vocational assessment process.

A good vocational assessment should include the collection and analysis of information about a child's vocational aptitudes, skills, expressed interests, and occupational exploration history (volunteer experiences, part-time or summer employment, club activities). The collection of this information should also take into account the child's language, culture, and family.

A Level I vocational assessment is administered at the beginning of a child's transitional process and is based on the child's abilities, expressed interests, and needs. This Level I assessment may include the review of existing school information and the conduct of informal interviews. A Level II vocational assessment usually includes the administration of one or more formal vocational evaluations. A Level III vocational assessment usually involves the analysis of a child's success in a real or simulated work setting. This is usually reported by a job coach, employer, or vocational evaluator. The transitional process should not be used to limit a student's educational or career aspirations. Instead, it should allow districts to provide opportunities at an earlier age.

Level I Vocational Assessment

Level I takes a look at the child from a vocational perspective. A trained vocational evaluator or knowledgeable special education teacher should be designated to collect the Level I assessment data. The information gathered for analysis should include existing information from

➤ cumulative records

➤ student interviews

➤ parent/guardian and teacher interviews

➤ special education eligibility data

➤ a review of the child's aptitudes

➤ achievements

➤ interests

➤ behaviors

➤ occupational exploration activities

The informal student interview involved in a Level I assessment should consider the child's vocational interest, interpersonal relationship skills, and adaptive behavior.

Level II Vocational Assessment

A Level II assessment is based upon the analysis obtained from the Level I assessment. This may be recommended by the CSE at any time to determine the level of a student's vocational skills, aptitudes, and interests, but not before the age of 12. Use the same knowledgeable staff members who were involved in prior assessments. Collected data should include:

➤ writing

➤ learning styles

➤ interest inventory

➤ motor (dexterity, speed, tool use, strength, coordination)

➤ spatial discrimination

➤ verbal reading

➤ perception (visual/auditory/tactile)

➤ speaking numerical (measurement, money skills)

➤ comprehension (task learning, problem solving)

➤ attention (staying on task)

Level III Vocational Assessment

A Level III vocational assessment is a comprehensive vocational evaluation that focuses on real or simulated work experiences. This assessment is the basis for vocational counseling. Unlike the Level I and Level II assessments, a trained vocational evaluator should administer or supervise this level of assessment. Level III assessment options consist of:

➤ Vocational evaluations including aptitudes and interests that are compared to job performance to predict vocational success in specific areas. Work samples must be valid and reliable.

➤ Situational vocational assessments, which occur in real work settings. These on-the-job assessments consider what has been learned and how.

➤ Work-study assessments are progress reports from supervisors or mentors that provide information on the child's job performance. A standard observational checklist may be utilized.

If a student plans a postsecondary educational program, he or she may benefit from two types of assessments:

1. *General assessments of postsecondary education skills* are necessary to determine academic skills, critical thinking skills, requirements for reasonable accommodations, social behaviors, interpersonal skills, self-advocacy and self-determination skills, learning strategies, and time management or organizational skills. This information is usually obtained through consultation with peers or teachers, or a self-evaluation.

2. *Assessments specific to field of study or setting* are necessary to assess needs, in relation to daily living skills, that may be experienced in a classroom setting or on a college campus. The identification of additional skills that a child must plan for to be an effective member of a postsecondary educational setting includes some of the following:

   – dormitory living vs. commuting

   – lab work

   – large lecture vs. seminar courses

Parents may wish to visit campuses that provide supportive services for children with disabilities. Information regarding colleges that provide these services can be obtained in local libraries, bookstores, or high school guidance offices.

Confidentiality

To bring the expertise of community-based nonschool personnel into the transitional planning process, the matter of confidentiality must be addressed. Under the Family Education Rights and Privacy Act (FERPA), aka Buckley Amendment, parents' rights to confidentiality must be maintained. During the transition process, families must sign releases, giving written consent, in order to benefit from available community resources. This does not commit a parent or the child to a specific service if at a later date it is not wanted or needed. Parents must ask their district about the rules of confidentiality regarding the release of information, the use of information by community agencies, and the storage of information once it is released by the district.

SPECIFIC PROFESSIONALS TRAINED TO HELP PARENTS AND THEIR CHILDREN PLAN AND PREPARE FOR EMPLOYMENT

There are a variety of people who are specifically trained to support students in planning and preparing for employment or other postsecondary school options. These people may include

➤ vocational counselors

➤ special and regular educators

➤ counselors from the Department of Rehabilitation Services (DRS)

➤ county case managers

PREVOCATIONAL SKILLS

If families have been properly advised through earlier stages of the transition process, their children should have learned job-related skills and behaviors, or prevocational skills, that can be fostered to help each child be successful in future employment. Examples of these skills include

➤ physical stamina

➤ promptness

➤ problem solving

➤ hygiene

➤ ability to follow directions

➤ independence in completing assigned tasks

➤ ability to establish social relationships with co-workers

Upon graduation from high school or the end of secondary school eligibility, the student will be faced with several options, depending upon the nature and severity of his or her disability. Many individuals with disabilities choose to pursue continued employment training in a postsecondary institution while others choose to begin working right away. This direction usually follows along with the student's vocational education plan, sometimes referred to as the transitional individual educational plan, that was developed while he or she was still in high school. This comprehensive plan should have assisted the student in developing the skills needed to find and keep a job after graduation. Schools may offer a vocational work experience with a job coach. In some schools, a student may have been assigned to a vocationally licensed teacher who operated as the work experience coordinator within the job site. If a school does not have such an individual, then a special education teacher would be responsible for developing the student's vocational goals.

While the student is still in school, the vocational counselor or individual assigned to develop a vocational plan begins to observe and develop a general transition checklist of possible vocational skills. These general observations may change from year to year as the student matures or they may remain the same because of the nature of the disability. Whatever the case, these observations are the beginning of what will be defined as vocational skills and needs. A sample checklist follows. This is not intended to be comprehensive but merely a beginning tool in assessing the student's needs and skills.

SKILLS CHECKLIST

Domestic Skills

Can the student

____ prepare a breakfast

____ prepare a lunch

____ prepare a supper

____ prepare a snack

____ pack his or her own lunch

_____ clean own room

_____ clean own apartment

_____ do own laundry

_____ use a washer or dryer

_____ make own meal plans

_____ budget his or her own time

Vocational Skills

Can the student

_____ get to/from work on time

_____ punch/sign in appropriately

_____ perform work satisfactorily

_____ work cooperatively with co-workers

_____ take break/lunch appropriately

_____ wear suitable clothing

_____ use appropriate safety measures

_____ follow directions

_____ accept supervision

Recreation/Leisure Skills

Can the student

_____ use free time for pleasure

_____ choose reasonable activities

_____ pick a hobby

_____ perform required activities

_____ use community resources

Community Skills

Can the student

_____ use public transportation

_____ shop for groceries

_____ shop for clothing

_____ make necessary appointments

_____ use the phone

_____ use bank accounts

_____ be safe in traffic

_____ respond appropriately to strangers

_____ know how to seek help

_____ handle money

Social/Personal Skills

Can the student

____ supply appropriate personal identification, if necessary

____ greet people appropriately

____ use contemporary style of dress, hair style, makeup

____ use good grooming/hygiene

____ "communicate" with friends/co-workers

____ be courteous and friendly

BASIC SERVICES RECEIVED THROUGH HIGH SCHOOL

The basic services students should have received during high school are:

➤ A vocational assessment of their interests and abilities

➤ Special services, including curriculum modifications that facilitate success in vocational programs

➤ Guidance, career counseling, and career development opportunities

➤ Counseling services to ease the transition from school to work

DIVISION OF REHABILITATION SERVICES (DRS)

At this point, it is necessary to seek out a counselor from the Division of Rehabilitation Services (DRS) located within your state. These services are usually well known to school counselors, who should have a brochure that is put out by this agency.

The counselor from DRS will work with the school, parents, and the student to help plan for employment needs. DRS primarily serves adults or individuals who have graduated or aged out from secondary education. It is important to involve the counselor during the transition process, however, so when the student graduates and enters the work force, the supports are in place that will allow him or her to be successfully employed.

To receive services from DRS, the student must meet certain requirements:

➤ The student must have a documented physical or mental disability that presents difficulties, or barriers to employment.

➤ There must be a good chance that DRS services will help him or her get and keep a job.

If the student is still being provided public school assistance, then the school will usually make an appointment for DRS involvement somewhere in the transitional process. If the student has more severe limitations, a DRS counselor can become involved during the very early stages of the planning. Also keep in mind that DRS services are time limited. For example, the agency will

➤ provide job-placement services

➤ ensure that the student with disabilities is satisfactorily employed

➤ provide follow-up services for at least 60 days and up to 18 months after the initial job placement

Files can be reopened if the student needs assistance to retain his or her current employment, find a new job, or reestablish a vocational program.

When a DRS agency is contacted, a VR (vocational rehabilitation) counselor will be assigned to work closely with the student and the family. The VR counselor will ask for background information that will help him or her work with the student. Questions usually focus on the following:

➢   goals

➢   interests

➢   educational history

➢   work history

➢   financial situation

➢   physical and emotional health

With parental permission the counselor may want to collect information from the student's doctor, hospital, or school, or to ask for evaluations at the expense of the DRS agency. The purpose of this gathering process is to give the counselor information about how the student's disability affects his or her ability to work and to help the counselor decide whether the student is eligible for services.

Services Provided by DRS Agencies

Based upon all available information, the DRS counselor will plan a program along with the family. Depending on what the student needs to meet his or her vocational goal, he or she may receive one or more of the following services that the agency buys and provides:

1.   A vocational assessment to help identify
     –   skills, abilities, and interests
     –   possible job goals
     –   services necessary to get a job and live as independently as possible

2.   A physical and/or psychological examination to help understand how the student's disability affects his or her ability to work

3.   Guidance, counseling, and referral to help the student with problems he or she may have

4.   Vocational counseling and career planning

5.   Short-term medical intervention to improve the student's ability to work (if not covered by family insurance)

6.   Training to learn the skills the student will need for the job he or she wants to enter, which may include
     –   on-the-job training
     –   job coach services
     –   college and university programs
     –   trade and business school programs
     –   personal adjustment programs
     –   work adjustment programs

7. Transition services

8. Driver evaluation and training

9. Homemaker evaluation and training

10. Services that may assist the student during assessment or training, including:
    - special transportation
    - some maintenance expenses
    - attendants, note takers, and interpreters
    - reader's aid for matriculated students

11. Supported employment (more on this later in the chapter)

12. Books, tools, and equipment that may be needed for training or employment

13. Telecommunications aids and adaptive devices that may be needed for employment

14. Assistance with some costs of modifications needed for employment
    - work site modifications
    - van or other vehicle modifications
    - home modifications

15. Training in job-seeking skills to learn how to
    - fill out a job application or develop a résumé
    - handle job interviews successfully
    - develop other job-related skills

16. Occupational licenses, tools, initial stock, and supplies for a small business

17. Job placement services to help the student find suitable work

18. Follow-up services to make sure of job satisfaction and deal with any problems relating to work

19. Referral to independent living services for
    - peer counseling
    - advice on other benefits
    - housing assistance
    - training in independent living skills

20. Assistance in working with agencies such as the
    - Social Security Administration
    - Department of Social Services
    - Office of Mental Health
    - Veterans Administration

Keep in mind that there is no guarantee that all agencies will pay for or provide all of these services. Investigate the agency in your particular community. While there is usually no cost for such services, sponsorship for some services may be based on the individual's income and/or family resources.

Following are the rights one has when involved with DRS services:

➤ To have the student's eligibility for VR services determined in a timely way regardless of age, color, religion, creed, disability, marital status, national origin, sexual orientation, or gender

➤ If eligible, to take part in planning vocational goals and the services needed to reach these goals

➤ If eligible, to receive services to reach his or her vocational goal

➤ To have goals tailored to his or her personal needs

➤ To receive an individual written rehabilitation program (IWRP)

➤ To have all information kept confidential

➤ To be informed of all decisions and actions of the DRS related to the case

➤ To be informed of rights as a consumer of DRS services

➤ To request and receive a timely review if there is any dissatisfaction with any actions or decisions by the DRS staff

Along with the student, families will have their own responsibilities if they get involved in DRS services. Families play an important role in working toward a successful outcome with the student. Both have the responsibility to

➤ Work closely with the DRS counselor to provide all information needed to plan a program.

➤ Ask questions if they don't understand any aspect of the program.

➤ Keep in touch with the counselor by letter or telephone. If the family moves, let the counselor know your new address and telephone number.

➤ Participate fully in developing an individual written rehabilitation program.

➤ Make every effort to identify and apply for sources of funding that will help pay for the vocational rehabilitation program.

➤ Help the child maintain satisfactory performance and regular attendance, whether in a training program or in a job.

➤ Let the counselor know, on a regular basis, how well the child is doing or what problems there are with the program.

➤ Work with the counselor to look for job openings and go on interviews when the student is ready for work.

➤ Let the counselor know if the student becomes employed. For at least two months after the child is employed, maintain contact with the counselor to let him or her know how things are working out and whether assistance of any kind is needed.

Conflict Resolution Options With DRS

Applying for DRS services is not a guarantee of eligibility. Many factors are considered, and each case is very different. If there is a rejection for services, or a need to resolve disagreements or concerns the family has about DRS services, ask for a review of the case. There are a variety of ways in which disagreements or concerns can be resolved as quickly as possible. Any individual—a lawyer or a relative—may represent you at this meeting. The options include:

➤ **Informal Meeting.** Parents meet with the child's counselor, his or her supervisor, and a representative, and try to resolve problems quickly and informally.

➤ **Administrative Review.** Parents can ask for a review by a district office manager. They must ask for this review, in writing, within 90 days of the decision or action, unless they have a good reason for waiting longer than 90 days.

➤ **Impartial Hearing.** Parents can ask for a formal hearing before an impartial hearing officer who does not work for DRS. They must ask for a hearing, in writing, within 90 days of the decision or action, unless they have a good reason for waiting longer than 90 days.

OTHER ASSESSMENT OPTIONS DURING THE VOCATIONAL TRANSITION PHASE

Functional Assessments

The purpose of completing a functional assessment is to identify the student's work characteristics, and training and support needs in relation to actual job requirements. Functional assessment information is gathered so that the best job match can be determined for an individual. The information must be interpreted in relation to the actual requirements of the job.

A functional assessment considers a wide variety of individual work characteristics including:

➤ availability to work

➤ transportation

➤ strength—lifting and carrying

➤ endurance

➤ physical mobility

➤ independent work rate

➤ appearance

➤ communication

➤ social skills

➤ unusual behaviors

➤ attention to task

➤ motivation

➤ adaptability to change

➤ reinforcement needs

➤ family support

➤ financial situation

➤ discrimination skills

➤ time awareness

➤ functional reading

➤ functional math

➤ independent street crossing

➤ ability to handle criticism

➤ ability to handle stress

➤ aggressive actions or speech

➤ travel skills

➤ benefits needed

The rehabilitation counselor, job placement specialist, or employment specialist can use the information from the functional assessment to identify a job in the community with requirements that match the skills, interests, and support needs of the student.

Keep in mind that vocational or situational assessments are recommended only when there is a need to

➤ determine whether the student is an appropriate candidate for supported employment

➤ identify the intensity of support services that he or she will need

➤ clarify inconsistent available information

➤ enhance insufficient information that is required to determine his or her employment needs

Situational Vocational Assessment

A situational assessment offers a person with a severe disability the opportunity to perform job tasks in real work environments in the community. Usually, a situational assessment is conducted for a four-hour period in three different types of jobs in the community where the service provider has established a working relationship with the employer. It is important that the jobs selected are representative of the types of jobs found in the local business community, for example, dishwasher, groundskeeper, grocery clerk.

The information obtained on the student during a situational assessment can assist in identifying the following characteristics about a potential worker:

➤ whether support is needed

➤ the type of support needed

➤ individual training needs and effective strategies

➤ the anticipated level of intervention

➤ the least restrictive environment

➤ other information needed to develop an appropriate individual written rehabilitation program

Actual performance in a job with appropriate training and support is the best predictor of an individual's performance in a supported employment situation. Observing an individual perform real work in multiple environments will provide an indication of the student's work characteristics, interests, skills, abilities, and training needs. For example:

➤ Does the student seem to show a preference across job types?

➤ Does the student work more effectively at specific times of the day?

➤ Does the student respond positively or negatively to factors in the environment—noise, movement, objects, people, amount of space, and so on?

➤ What types of prompts does the student respond to and what is the frequency?

WHO CONDUCTS A SITUATIONAL ASSESSMENT?

Situational assessments can be requested from a supported employment vendor or a vocational evaluator. The purpose of such an assessment must be to determine the appropriateness of supported employment and the extent of supported employment services needed.

WHAT INFORMATION SHOULD YOU EXPECT TO RECEIVE AFTER THE SITUATIONAL ASSESSMENT IS COMPLETED?

It is important to obtain a written report from the vendor who completes the situational assessment. The report should include

➤ a description of the jobs completed

➤ the behavioral data obtained during the assessment process

➤ a summary of the student's characteristics

TRAINING AND WORK OPTIONS

Once the assessment is complete, the student will be presented with a variety of training and work options, depending upon the results of the evaluation. Many options and directions are available.

Internships and Apprenticeships

Internships are similar to on-the-job training. They are time-limited, paid or unpaid jobs that permit the intern to sample the type of work available in a general field. Many high school and community transition programs offer individuals the opportunity to participate in an internship prior to competitive employment. By participating in an internship, individuals can learn more about the job and have the opportunity to familiarize themselves with the work environment.

Apprenticeship programs have been a historical means of preparing competent and skilled workers. Apprenticeships offer individuals the opportunity to learn the skills necessary for an occupation by working under the supervision of experienced workers. These programs generally take from three to four years to complete, but participants are paid for their labor. In the beginning, wages may not be more than minimum wage, but by the end of the program, wages are usually nearly those earned by an experienced worker. Generally, the sponsor of the apprenticeship is a company or a group of companies, a public agency, or a union. Over 700 organizations are currently involved in apprenticeship programs.

Local unions, vocational education programs in the community, the state office of vocational rehabilitation, and the state employment office are all sources of more information about apprenticeship opportunities. Each state also has a state occupational informational coordinating committee (overseen at the federal level by the National Occupational Informational Coordinating Committee). These committees, to differing degrees in each state, provide systems for individuals to obtain information about apprenticeships. The Bureau of Apprenticeship and Training also has regional offices throughout the United States. To locate the office serving your area, write or call the Bureau of Apprenticeship and Training, 200 Constitution Avenue N.W., Washington, DC 20210, (202)535-0540.

TRAINING OFFERED BY DISABILITY-SPECIFIC ORGANIZATIONS

Organizations such as ARC (formerly the Association for Retarded Citizens), the United Cerebral Palsy Foundation (UCPF), and others serving people with a specific disability may provide vocational assessment and training. The types of training provided vary, but the goals of the training are that individuals with disabilities will obtain employment and become as independent as possible. As an example, many regional offices of ARC provide training in computer skills and other office skills to persons with mental retardation who have been referred to the ARC program. This training often leads to competitive employment for these individuals.

To find out more about disability-specific organizations operating in your state or local area, contact NICHCY for a state resource sheet.

ADULT EDUCATION

Adult education programs are designed to provide instruction below the college level to any person age 16 or older who is no longer being served by the public education system. There are many different programs available, and you can find them in a variety of settings. One setting of importance to youth seeking vocational training is an area vocational center. In many states, area vocational centers operate as part of the public school system. Secondary school students may receive vocational instruction in the area vocational center during the day, while instruction for adults in the community would generally be available there at night. Vocational courses may include training in such areas as health care, business education, home economics, industrial arts, marketing, or trades such as carpentry or automotive mechanics. The course of study might involve students in apprenticeships (discussed above), which can lead to certification in a trade or recognized occupation. Adult education programs may also be available to prepare individuals for GED (General Equivalency Diploma) tests or to teach English as a Second Language (ESL). Continuing education programs may also be offered under the auspices of adult education; however, continuing education is generally meant to provide personal enrichment rather than vocational training. For example, continuing education classes may be offered in areas such as cooking, gardening, or sewing.

Information about adult education programs—whether they are intended as vocational training or personal enrichment—can usually be obtained by contacting your local education agency.

TRADE AND TECHNICAL SCHOOLS

These schools are designed to prepare students for gainful employment in recognized occupations. Examples include occupations such as air conditioning technician, bank teller, cosmetologist, dental assistant, data processor, electrician, medical secretary, surveyor, and welder. Vocational training is provided so that an individual can obtain skills in a specific area of interest or increase the level of skills he or she has already achieved. A course of study may take anywhere from two weeks to two years to complete, with the general entrance requirement of a GED or high school diploma. These schools typically place great importance on job placement for their graduates. If students are working with a high school counselor or a vocational counselor at the VR office in or near their community, one of these schools may be recommended to them as a way of getting the training they need.

COMPETITIVE EMPLOYMENT

Competitive employment can be defined as full-time or part-time jobs in the open labor market with competitive wages and responsibilities. Competitive employment is employment that the individual maintains with no more outside support than a co-worker without a disability would receive. The key word here is *maintains*. Although a student may make use of transition services available in the community in order to prepare for and find competitive employment, these services are temporary. Once the individual has the job, support from outside agencies is terminated, and the individual maintains, or does, the job on his or her own.

The types of jobs that are normally considered competitive employment are as vast in number as they are varied. Waitresses, service station attendants, clerks, secretaries, mechanics, professional drivers, factory workers, computer programmers and managers, teacher's aides, teachers, health care workers, lawyers, scientists, and engineers are just some examples of people who are competitively employed. As can be seen by these examples, the amount of training an individual needs varies considerably from job to job. Some jobs are entry level and require little or no specific training. Other jobs require vocational preparation and training, while still others require extensive academic schooling.

Recently, a training model known as *transitional employment* has been useful in helping many young people prepare for competitive employment. Transitional employment is aimed at those individuals who cannot enter into competitive work on their own. With training and support, however, they may be able to handle a full wage job. Among those who have benefited from transitional employment are individuals who are mentally disabled, learning disabled, or developmentally disabled, and persons with hearing and vision impairments.

The important thing to remember about competitive employment, however, is that the assistance and supports offered by a human services agency are time-limited in nature and end once the student has secured employment.

SUPPORTED EMPLOYMENT

Two aspects must be considered when confronted with vocational decisions—finding a job and keeping a job. The student may require little or no help with one or both aspects, or he or she may require a great deal of help. As we have seen, help with finding a job comes from the school system, in partnership with the vocational rehabilitation agency.

Employment in which a student will need long-term or ongoing help to keep a job is called supported employment. Supported employment is a job with pay at a business in the community. Supported employment is for adults who

➤ traditionally have not been considered part of the workforce

➤ need long-term support to be employed

➤ have one or more disabilities, such as mental retardation, autism, mental illness, traumatic brain injury, physical disabilities, severe learning disabilities, or severe behavioral challenges

➤ require intensive, repetitive, or adaptive assistance to learn new tasks

How Do Parents Know If Their Children Need Supported Employment?

If a child is already involved in a work situation or has been involved in the past, you should be aware of several signals that may indicate the need for supported employment services. These include, but are not limited to,

➤ repeated failures to maintain employment without support

➤ failure or inability to generalize skills from preemployment training programs

➤ problems acquiring skills

➤ significant communication problems where job-site advocacy would help social integration with co-workers and supervisors

➤ the need for extended training and support to develop production rates.

Help for the child is provided by the same companies that specialize in finding employment for adults with disabilities. They can provide a job coach to give help directly to the child with disabilities. Optimally, the job coach will train the child's co-workers and supervisors to provide the supports that are needed to maintain his or her effectiveness on the job. Other services that are provided by job coaches include

➤ travel training

➤ task analysis

➤ hands-on instruction

➤ developing job-modification accommodations

➤ developing visual or other tools to improve productivity

➤ training in appropriate job behaviors

➤ developing natural supports and social skills

➤ employee liaison problem solving

➤ parent liaison

➤ advocate for employee with disability

The amount and kind of help that is provided to find and keep a job should be based on the needs and abilities of the student with disabilities. When a parent is involved with an agency that will provide employment services for the child, the parent will need to learn as much as possible about the agency in order to assess its ability to meet the child's vocational needs and goals. Therefore, parents should ask the following questions:

1. What types of jobs are available?

2. How does the agency select a job for an individual with disabilities?

3. Where are the actual job locations?

4. Does the agency provide individual or group placements?

5. How does the agency promote integration?

6. What are the average wages of employees?

7. What is the average number of hours worked per week?

8. What type of support does the agency provide?

9. Is transportation provided? What type, and by whom?

10. What are the average benefit packages available to employees?

11. What provisions does the agency have for employee and parent or family input?

Supported employment is a major avenue to inclusion of persons with disabilities in their communities. As a service, it also reflects the growing conviction by persons with disabilities and their families that they have the right to be involved in decisions affecting the quality of their lives.

While the transition from high school to adult life is a complex time for all students, it can be especially challenging for young people with disabilities. The goal of parents and professionals is to help the child make this transition to the world of work as easily as possible. Being informed and educated as to options, rights, and resources can only enhance the child's transition into the vocational phase of his or her life.

SHELTERED WORKSHOPS

In sheltered employment options, individuals with disabilities work in a self-contained unit; they are not integrated with workers who do not have disabilities. Sheltered employment options typically range along a continuum from adult day programs to work activity centers to sheltered workshops. In adult day programs, individuals generally receive training in daily living skills, social skills, recreational skills, and prevocational skills. Work activity centers offer individuals similar training but may also include training in vocational skills. In sheltered workshops, individuals perform subcontracted tasks such as sewing, packaging, collating, or machine assembly and are usually paid on a piece-rate basis. Typically, people do not advance to the workshop until they have demonstrated certain mastery levels. Sheltered employment options are generally supported by federal and/or state funds and are operated by private, nonprofit corporations governed by a volunteer board of directors.

Traditionally, sheltered employment options were thought to be the only options available for individuals with severe disabilities. There is now evidence from supported employment models that individuals with severe disabilities can work in community settings if provided with adequate support. With the emergence of supported employment, many facilities began to modify their sheltered employment programs to provide workers with integrated options. Advocates of this trend away from sheltered employment point to the advantages of supported employment, which include higher wages, more meaningful work, and integration with workers who do not have disabilities.

OTHER AVENUES TO EMPLOYMENT

There are many avenues that lead to stable, satisfying employment. This section addresses other avenues a young person with a disability can take to employment—learning and growing along the way. For young people with disabilities, early job experiences are vital learning situations wherein they gain good work habits such as punctuality, responsibility, insight into appropriate behaviors, and standards of personal grooming. As such, initial jobs need not *always* place the individual on a career ladder. Sometimes it is useful to take jobs as stepping stones in one's training, rather than as the final step in employment. Temporary work can be one such stepping stone. Employers often have trouble finding a person to take a job that will last only several weeks or months. For a young person with a disability, a temporary job may offer the opportunity to get valuable work experience, earn wages, and develop a work history. Part-time work is a similar stepping stone in many ways. Part-time employment offers many advantages for persons who need to attend school part of the day, or who may be uncertain as to their work stamina or tolerance. Job-sharing is another stepping stone, where two workers share the responsibilities of one full-time job. All of these examples can offer individuals meaningful employment that suits their schedule or their mental or physical abilities. These are also excellent ways by which to enter an organization, establish a reputation as a worker, and possibly move into a full-time job when one becomes available or is desired.

Programs also exist that are designed to provide experience outside of a traditional classroom, for example, volunteering and international exchange programs. Both types of programs offer personal enrichment to young adults and enhance their independence, self-advocacy skills, and their ability to make informed choices about further education and careers.

Volunteering

Volunteering enables a student or adult with a disability to develop a work history and can lead to paid employment. Some transition programs provide opportunities for young adults with disabilities to have volunteer experiences in several career areas as part of career exploration and selection. A volunteer organization in your community, county, or state may also be able to provide you with information about volunteer opportunities. At the national level, VOLUNTEER: The National Center for Citizen Involvement has been developing projects on the use of volunteers who have disabilities; this organization may be able to provide information specific to your locality. Contact VOLUNTEER at P.O. Box 1807, Boulder, CO 80306. Also at the national level is AmeriCorps, a federal agency that runs the VISTA program (Volunteers in Service to America). VISTA can be contacted, toll-free, at (800)424-8867 for information on recruitment and current projects, as well as information about state and regional offices. The number for AmeriCorps is (800)94-ACORPS.

International Exchange Programs

International exchange programs can also serve as stepping stones for young people with disabilities. While the programs cannot be considered employment, they nevertheless are personally enriching and, for a young person with a disability, lead to increased independence. There are two general types of international exchange programs: educational exchanges and international workcamps. Educational exchange programs enable young adults to live, study, or volunteer in another country while living with a host family or with other participants in a dormitory. International workcamps bring persons with disabilities and persons without disabilities together to work on community projects in host countries. Individuals with disabilities have participated successfully in both kinds of international programs. For more information about exchange programs, contact Mobility International USA, P.O. Box 10767, Eugene, OR 97440, (503)343-1284 (Voice/TDD) or The U.S. Committee of the International Christian Youth Exchange (ICYE), 134 West 26th Street, New York, NY 10001, (212)206-7307.

The Military

The military may also be a viable postsecondary option for many young adults with disabilities. Some individuals with learning disabilities, for example, can benefit from the highly structured, repetitive, and physically active regime of military life. To pursue a career in the military, however, individuals must meet the qualifications of the specific branch of interest. The student or parent should talk to a recruiter in the particular branch of interest prior to graduation in order to find out about requirements. It is also important to know that Section 504 of the Rehabilitation Act does not cover uniformed personnel branches of the military; therefore, no particular accommodations are made regarding a person's disability unless that person is a civilian employee.

Civilian Service in Military Installations

There are also opportunities for civilian service employees in military installations. The majority of these positions are in an administrative or support-staff capacity. These provide opportunities for persons skilled in the areas of accounting, computer technology, contracting, and clerical duties. The best avenue for a person with a disability to take in order to obtain employment as a civilian is to be certified by the Vocational Rehabilitation System for Schedule A employment. The person may then apply directly to the federal government agency in which he or she is interested, including military installations around the nation and the world. Each installation in the military has to adhere to equal opportunity standards for employees in civilian positions.

Entrepreneurship

Entrepreneurship is a nontraditional avenue many individuals with disabilities have taken to employment. Rather than work for someone else, they decided to start a business of their own. For some persons, the focus of the business grew out of a hobby or a personal interest. An example of this is Don Krebs, who became a quadriplegic as a result of a water-skiing accident. After his recovery, Don searched for adaptive equipment to allow him to return to water-skiing, a sport he loved, and in the process recognized the great need for adaptive recreation equipment. Using money from SSDI and his Plan for Achieving Self Support (PASS), Don started Access to Recreation, a mail-order company specializing in adaptive recreation equipment.

BUSINESS OPPORTUNITIES

Some individuals with disabilities who have successfully created their own business began with the desire to work out of their homes. Betty, for instance, is mobility-impaired and uses a wheelchair. She operates a direct mail order business from her home and sells eyeglass frames wholesale to optometrists and opticians.

Other people with disabilities have become involved in businesses their parents have created. Laura and Charles, for example, have a son who is severely mentally retarded. Concerned about Harold's employment prospects, Laura and Charles joined forces several years ago with two other families whose children are mentally retarded. Together, the parents purchased ten vending machines which they then situated in strategic locations. The young adults, who now range in age from 18 to 25, are responsible for tending to the machines—restocking them with sodas, retrieving the coins and rolling them up for deposit in the bank, and reporting any machine malfunctions to their parents. Although it took the families several months to identify the most lucrative spots to place the vending machines, the amount of income generated by this small business has surprised them all.

STARTING AND MAINTAINING A BUSINESS

Starting and maintaining a business is a serious enterprise. The ingenuity, determination, and stamina of participants are important factors in producing success or failure. Operating a small business can offer many advantages to individuals with disabilities, however, such as minimizing transportation concerns, setting one's own work hours, and having the freedom to modify the job in whatever way is necessary to get the job done most efficiently, given the personality and disability of the individual. Persons interested in starting a business can contact the Small Business Administration for assistance and advice. SBA can also help you secure a loan through a bank or other commercial lender. SBA operates more than 100 local offices across the country. To find out if an office exists in your vicinity, consult your telephone directory or contact the SBA central office at 409 3rd Street, S.W., Information Center, Room 100, Washington, DC 20416, (202)606-4000 (in the DC area) or (800)827-5722.

JOB SEARCH METHODS

(The remaining sections of this chapter are addressed to the young person who will be engaged in the job search—with assistance as needed from parents and professionals.)

People look for jobs for many different reasons: they are laid off, they want to reenter the work force, they want or need to relocate, they dislike their present job, they want to get a better job, or they are entering the labor force for the first time. This section provides guidelines for preparing for and conducting a job search. Steps discussed include

➤   developing a résumé

➤   locating prospective employers

➤ applying for the job

➤ interviewing

➤ following through

These are only guidelines; you will find additional detailed information at your public library, or at high school or college career centers.

Developing a Résumé

The two main types of résumés are the chronological and the functional. A chronological résumé is used when you have had a fairly direct path of development from one position to another in the same field. A functional résumé emphasizes your skills, and is used by people who change jobs or careers frequently. A good résumé will be one page long and will capture your career goals, and education and work history. For some positions, you may have to include a sample of your writing.

A résumé should include the following information:

➤ name

➤ address

➤ telephone number

➤ job objective or career goal

➤ educational history (degrees, certificates, courses, accomplishments)

➤ work history, including military service (skills, experience), and memberships related to your job objective

Depending on the position for which you are applying, it might also include work-related honors or achievements, knowledge of foreign languages, ability to travel or relocate, and security clearance information.

Job Application Forms

Some jobs do not require a formal résumé but may call for a written application. Most application forms require such basic information as

➤ name

➤ address and telephone number

➤ social security number

➤ dates of previous jobs

➤ names and addresses of former employers and

➤ dates of schooling or training

Before you begin to fill out the application, read it through to be sure that you have all required information. It is very important that you print the information neatly and legibly. If your application makes a poor impression, you are unlikely to go further with that employer.

Although not every job calls for letters of reference, you should ask people if they would be willing to write one for you. Do not list someone as a reference unless you have his or her permission to do so. Candidates for references include former employers, teachers, volunteer supervisors, and other people who can assess your character.

Locating Employers

When you have determined the kind of job you want, you must locate potential employers. Among the most frequently used methods of finding them are making "cold calls"; getting information from friends, relatives, or colleagues; reading want ads; and using employment agencies. Usually, more than one source will be used and there are advantages and disadvantages to all methods.

"COLD CALLS"

This technique involves visiting employers to see if there are openings. A person using this method of finding a job needs high motivation and good interpersonal skills. Sometimes, talking directly to the person who makes the hiring decision rather than the personnel office produces better results. Before calling on small companies, it is a good idea to call or write ahead of time; they may not appreciate interruptions. Letters, followed by phone calls, can be effective for small and medium-sized businesses. Advantages of cold calls are that some jobs are not listed anywhere, the opening may be new, and you may be in the right place at the right time. Disadvantages include the time involved and the high rejection rate.

NETWORKING

Learning about an opening through friends, relatives, or co-workers is the most successful way to get a job; most employers do not like to hire strangers. They know that people who are referred to a company tend to be more stable and therefore will stay longer in the job. Advantages of networking are that referrals often guarantee an interview, jobs offered often are better with higher pay, and it is easier to develop a relationship with the potential employer when referred by a colleague.

NEWSPAPER ADS

Many people start their job search with want ads. This is unfortunate because it is frequently a last resort for employers. Advantages of classified ads are that they list specific openings and have frequent new listings. Disadvantages are that the jobs are often undesirable or hard to fill, or have a high turnover rate; positions are often at the high and low ends of the skill/experience spectrum—few in the middle; there is little information about the job or employer; competition is intense; and ads list a small proportion of available jobs.

EMPLOYMENT AGENCIES

Public employment services are funded by the federal government and administered by states. They are widely viewed as ineffective, primarily offering low-paying, low-status jobs. Their main advantage is that there is no cost to the client or employer. Disadvantages are that they are usually looking for unskilled or casual labor, there are fewer occupations offered than are listed in want ads, and they offer limited opportunities.

Private or temporary agencies will, for a fee, try to match employers and employees. Depending on the agency and the position offered, the fee may be paid entirely by the employer or by the employee, or they may split it. Some agencies specialize in a particular field such as clerical work or sales. Private agencies tend to be more successful with experienced people who have sharply defined skills, good work histories, and employment in a single field. Advantages are that they offer a chance for employer and prospective employee to explore the possibility of a permanent relationship, and they may list positions not offered elsewhere. The main disadvantage is the fee.

Applying and Interviewing for Jobs

Once you have found a job that sounds good to you, you must apply for it. This involves writing to the company offering the job and including your résumé or a job application. In either case, your cover letter is very important; it is the first thing that your prospective employer will see. The letter should be personalized and contain information such as where you heard about the job, an indication of your interest, why you are suited for the position, and your interest in interviewing. It should include your name, address, and phone number.

The next step in the job search is the job interview, which involves an exchange between people trying to find out whether they can work together to mutual benefit. Before you go to the interview, learn as much as you can about a prospective employer by reading brochures, talking to present employees, calling the chamber of commerce, or visiting the public library. Some interviewing dos and don'ts: *do* be honest; be prompt (better ten minutes early than one minute late); use a firm handshake; dress appropriately; make eye contact; address interviewer by name—pronounced correctly; use good grammar; know something about the company; prepare to ask intelligent and thoughtful questions; *don't* sound arrogant; be too personal; smoke or chew gum; make excuses; bring up salary at the first interview.

After the interview, it is important to maintain contact with the prospective employer. Write a thank-you letter, indicating that you will call at a specific time to find out your status regarding the position. Call when you said you would. If the answer is no, ask why. Knowing why you did not get a job may help you get the next one.

YOUR EMPLOYMENT RIGHTS IN THE PRIVATE SECTOR

Disabilities and Job Discrimination

Individuals with disabilities are protected from discrimination in employment primarily by two federal laws. The Americans With Disabilities Act (P.L. 101-336), enacted into law on July 26, 1990, prohibits private sector employers who employ fifteen or more individuals and all state and local government employers from discriminating against qualified individuals with disabilities in all aspects of employment.

The Rehabilitation Act of 1973 (P.L. 93-112), as amended, prohibits discrimination in employment in three areas.

REHABILITATION ACT: SECTION 501

Section 501 of the Rehabilitation Act prohibits federal executive branch agencies, including the U.S. Postal Service and the Postal Rate Commission, from discriminating against qualified individuals with disabilities. It requires executive branch agencies to take affirmative action in the hiring, placing, and advancing of individuals with disabilities.

REHABILITATION ACT: SECTION 503

Section 503 of the Rehabilitation Act requires contractors and subcontractors who have contracts with the federal government for $10,000 or more annually to take affirmative action to employ and to advance in employment qualified individuals with disabilities.

REHABILITATION ACT: SECTION 504

Section 504 prohibits recipients of federal financial assistance from discriminating against qualified individuals with disabilities in employment and in their programs and activities.

Title I: Employment and the ADA*

The Americans With Disabilities Act (ADA) 1990 is modeled after the Rehabilitation Act of 1973 and the Civil Rights Act of 1964. The purpose of the ADA is to assure civil rights protections to qualified people with disabilities. The ADA prohibits discrimination on the basis of disability in the private sector and in state and local government.

In addition to prohibitions against discrimination in employment, the ADA also prohibits discrimination in public accommodations and services, transportation provided by public and private entities, and in the provision of telecommunication services.

In terms of employment, the ADA requires nondiscrimination in all employment practices on the basis of disability, and specific actions to assure equal employment opportunity.

The ADA's employment provisions will ultimately cover all employers who have fifteen or more employees. Under the ADA, an employer may not discriminate against a person with a disability when the person is qualified to perform the essential functions of the job, with or without a reasonable accommodation.

According to the ADA, a *disabled individual* is one who has a documented physical or mental impairment which substantially limits a major life activity—walking, seeing, hearing, learning, caring for oneself. The ADA also defines a physical impairment as a physiological disorder or condition, cosmetic disfigurement, or anatomical loss; and a mental or psychological disorder as mental retardation, emotional or mental illness, or specific learning disabilities.

A *qualified individual* with a disability is protected under the ADA. A qualified individual with a disability as defined by the ADA is one who, with or without reasonable accommodation, can perform the essential functions of the job. An employer is required to make an accommodation to the known disability of a qualified applicant or employee if it would not impose an undue hardship on the operation of the employer's business.

Undue hardship is defined as an action requiring significant difficulty or expense when considered in light of factors such as the employer's size, financial resources, and the nature and structure of the operation.

Reasonable accommodation means that there is some modification in a job's tasks or structure, that is, making existing facilities used by employees readily accessible to and usable by persons with disabilities, in the workplace, which will allow the qualified employee with the disability to do the job. Employers also must make accommodations to enable people with disabilities to participate in the job application process and to enjoy benefits and privileges enjoyed by other employees. The modification or change must be made unless it would be an undue hardship for the employer.

---

* *Source:* Adapted from "Ready, Willing, and Available, A Business Guide for Hiring People With Disabilities," President's Committee on Employment of People With Disabilities, 8/93.

While employers are not permitted to ask applicants about the existence, nature, or severity of a disability, they may ask about the ability to perform specific job functions. If the applicant has a known disability that appears to interfere with or prevent job performance, the employer may ask the applicant to describe or demonstrate how he or she would do the job, with or without an accommodation.

A job offer may be conditioned on the results of a medical examination, but only if the examination is required for all entering employees in similar jobs. Medical examinations of current employees must be job related and consistent with business necessity. The results of all medical examinations and information from inquiries about a disability must be kept confidential, and maintained in separate medical files.

To file a complaint, contact the nearest EEOC (Equal Employment Opportunities Commission) office or call (800)669-4000 (Voice) or (800)800-3302 (TTY/TDD). If EEOC dismisses the complaint or fails to take action within 180 days, EEOC will issue the individual a right-to-sue letter, upon the person's request. The individual must sue within 90 days of the date of the notice.

Applicants or Employees With Disabilities in State or Local Government Agencies

If a state or local government employer employs fifteen or more people, an individual with a disability is covered by Title I of the ADA, enforced by the EEOC. A state or local government that employs fifteen or more employees is also covered by Title II of the ADA, which is enforced by the U.S. Department of Justice.

To file a complaint, contact the nearest EEOC office or call (800)669-4000 (Voice) or (800)800-3302 (TTY/TDD).

If a state or local government employer employs fewer than fifteen employees, an individual with a disability is covered by Title II of the ADA, enforced by the U.S. Department of Justice.

To file a complaint, send it to the U.S. Department of Justice, Civil Rights Division, Coordination and Review Section, P.O. Box 66118, Washington, DC, 20035-6118.

If a state or local employer receives federal financial assistance, an individual with a disability is also covered by Section 504 of the Rehabilitation Act of 1973, as amended, enforced by the federal agency that provided the federal financial assistance. The enforcement of Section 504 is coordinated by the U.S. Department of Justice.

To file a complaint, send it to the agency that provided the funds or to the U.S. Department of Justice, Civil Rights Division, Coordination and Review Section, P.O. Box 66118, Washington, DC, 20035-6118.

Individuals do not have to exhaust administrative procedures under Section 504 of the Rehabilitation Act. They may file suit against a public entity in federal district court, without filing a complaint with an administrative agency.

A FINAL WORD

A person who is able to work in any of the settings reviewed in this chapter must be actively involved in this phase of the transition process. This particular phase, probably more than most others, has long-term implications. Finding the right match between one's abilities and one's opportunities is often filled with many challenges, and therefore patience, fortitude, and flexibility are helpful assets.

— GLOSSARY —

accessible—easy to approach, enter, operate, participate in, or use safely and with dignity by a person with a disability (site, facility, work environment, service, or program).

adaptive behavior—make suitable or consistent with a particular situation or use.

affirmative action—positive action to accomplish the purposes of a program designed to increase the employment opportunities of certain groups, which may involve goals, timetables, or specifically outlined steps to be undertaken to assure that objectives are reached. The Americans With Disabilities Act does not mandate affirmative action for persons with disabilities, but does require that covered entities ensure nondiscrimination. Title 5, Section 503 of the Rehabilitation Act does require that affirmative action be taken in employment considerations of persons with disabilities by federal contractors.

aging out—the age at which a person with disabilities is no longer entitled to a free and appropriate education along with its supported services.

Americans With Disabilities Act (ADA)—A comprehensive civil rights law which makes it unlawful to discriminate in private-sector employment against a qualified individual with a disability. The ADA also outlaws discrimination against individuals with disabilities in state and local government services and employment, public accommodations, transportation, and telecommunication.

aptitudes—an inherent ability, as for learning, a talent

auxiliary aids and services—Devices or services that accommodate a functional limitation of a person with a communication disability. The term includes qualified interpreters and communication devices for persons who are deaf or hard of hearing; qualified readers, taped texts, Braille or other devices for persons with visual impairments; adaptive equipment or similar services and actions for persons with other communication disabilities.

competitive employment—generally defined as paid employment in a nonsheltered business or industry.

Equal Employment Opportunity (EEO)—nondiscrimination in hiring, firing, compensation, promotion, recruitment, training, and other terms and conditions of employment regardless of race, color, sex, age, religion, national origin or disability.

essential job functions—the fundamental job duties of the employment position that the individual with a disability holds or desires. The term *essential functions* does not include marginal functions of the position.

independent living services—nonprofit organizations that offer individuals with disabilities a variety of services and help individuals with disabilities to have more control over their lives and live more independently within the community. They are controlled by a board of directors, most of whom have disabilities themselves.

individual with a disability—a person who has a physical or mental impairment that substantially limits one or more of that person's major life activities, has a record of such impairment, or who is regarded as having such an impairment.

job coach—person who provides job training for a disabled worker in a competitive job location.

major life activity—basic activity that the average person in the general population can perform with little or no difficulty, including caring for self, performing manual tasks, walking, seeing, hearing, speaking, breathing, learning, and working.

prevocational skills—job-related skills and behaviors that are usually taught to individuals with disabilities prior to supported employment or some vocational setting.

qualified individual with a disability—an individual with a disability who satisfies the requisite skill, experience, education, and other job-related requirements of the employment position such individual holds or desires, and who, with or without reasonable accommodation, can perform the essential functions of such position.

reader's aide—a supportive assistant to an individual with a disability, who provides information that the disabled person may not be able to read.

reasonable accommodation—(1) modification or adjustment to a job application process that enables a qualified applicant with a disability to be considered for the position such qualified applicant desires; or (2) modifications or adjustments to the work environment, or to the manner or circumstances under which the position held or desired is customarily performed, that enables qualified individuals with disabilities to perform the essential functions of that position; or (3) modifications or adjustments that enable a covered entity's employee with a disability to enjoy benefits and privileges of employment equal to those enjoyed by its other similarly situated employees without disabilities.

sheltered workshop—a segregated place where work or samples of work are performed by people with disabilities; supervision, training, and vocational evaluation are provided by professional staff; wages are usually at a subminimum level.

supported employment—generally defined as paid employment in business or industry with job training and support services available as long as needed.

undue hardship—with respect to the provision of an accommodation, significant difficulty or expense incurred by a covered entity, when considered in light of certain factors. These factors include the nature and cost of the accommodation in relationship to the size, resources, nature, and structure of the employer's operation.

vocational evaluation—a battery of tests, some of which are standardized, to determine a disabled person's work skills and abilities.

— REFERENCES —

More information, including examples of application forms, résumés, cover and follow-up letters, and frequently asked interview questions will be found in high school and college career centers and at your public library. They also have materials directed to special populations such as veterans, minorities, and women. This bibliography lists examples of the types of materials you will find there. These will also assist you in writing résumés, getting interviews, developing contacts, establishing networks, marketing yourself, and writing cover letters.

Allen, J. 1994. *Successful Job Search Strategies for the Disabled: Understanding the ADA.* New York, John Wiley.

Allen, T. E., Rawlings, B. W., and Schildroth, A. 1989. *Deaf Students and the School-to-Work Transition.* Baltimore, MD: Paul H. Brookes.

Asher, D. 1995. *The Fool-Proof Job Search Workbook.* Ten Speed Press, Berkeley, CA.

Baxter, R., and Brashear, M. 1990. *Do-It-Yourself Career Kit—A Career Planning Tool.* Moraga, CA: Bridgewater Press. Step-by-step guidance in finding out about yourself and what you want from work, zeroing in on job opportunities, and getting where you want to go.

Beatty, Richard H. 1989. *The Perfect Cover Letter.* New York: John Wiley. Purpose and importance of cover letters, good and bad design, and practical advice regarding information to be included.

Berstein, A. 1996. *Guide to Your Career.* New York, Random House.

Big Book of Jobs. 1996. VGM Career Horizons. Lincolnwood, IL.

Bloch, D. P. 1992. *How to Have a Winning Job Interview.* Lincolnwood, IL: VGM Career Horizons. Offers 12 steps to a winning interview and helps you decide if the job for which you are interviewing is the one you want.

Bloch, D. P. 1989. *How to Write a Winning Résumé.* Lincoln, IL: VGM Career Horizons. A step-by-step guide to help you through the résumé-writing process.

Bloomfield, W. M. 1989. *Career Action Plan.* Bloomington, IL: Meridian Education Corporation. Exercises and activities that will help you plan your future as it relates to your career.

Bolles, R. 1992. *Job Hunting Tips for the So-Called Handicapped.* Special Needs Project, 1482 East Valley Rd., #A-121, Santa Barbara, CA 93108, (800)333-6867.

Bolles, R. 1996. *What Color Is Your Parachute?* Berkeley, CA: Ten Speed Press.

Brett. P. 1993. *Résumé Writing for Results.* Belmont, CA: Wadsworth Pub.

Calkins, C. F, and Walker, H. M. (eds.). 1990. *Social Competence for Workers With Developmental Disabilities.* Baltimore, MD: Paul H. Brookes.

Izzo, M. V., and Shumate, K. 1991. *Network for Effective Transitions to Work: A Transition Coordinator's Handbook.* Columbus, OH: Center for Education and Training for Employment. [Available from Center for Education and Training for Employment, Ohio State University, Publications Department, 1900 Kenny Road, Columbus, OH 43210-1090, Telephone: (800)848-4815.]

Jandt, F. 1996. *Using the Internet and the World Wide Web in Your Job Search.* Indianapolis, IN: JIST Works.

Kimeldorf, M. 1989. *Pathways to Work.* Bloomington, IL: Meridian Education Corporation. What employers look for in an application, what kinds of questions are asked during an interview, and how to describe your skills and interests.

Kimeldorf, M. 1990. *Write Into a Job.* Bloomington, IL: Meridian Education Corporation. How to write a résumé that will highlight your qualities.

Leach, L. N., and Harmon, A. S. 1991. *Annotated Bibliography on Transition From School to Work.* Champaign, IL: Transition Research Institute. [Available from Transition Research Institute at Illinois, College of Education, University of Illinois at Urbana-Champaign, 61 Childrens Research Center, 51 Gerty Drive, Champaign, IL 61820, Telephone: (217)333-2325.]

Moon, M. S.; Inge, K. J.; Wehman, P.; Brooke, V.; and Barcus, J. M. 1990. *Helping Persons With Severe Mental Retardation Get and Keep Employment: Supported Employment Strategies and Outcomes.* Baltimore, MD: Paul H. Brookes.

Passage, Your Workplace and Job Skills Information Newsletter. Information on all aspects of the job search. [Available from Beaver County Area Labor-Management Committee, 617 Midland Avenue, Midland, PA 15059.]

Powell, T. H.; Pancsofar, E. L.; Steer, D. E.; Butterworth, J.; Itzkowitz, J. S.; and Rainforth, B. 1991. *Supported Employment: Providing Integrated Employment Opportunities for Persons With Disabilities.* White Plains, NY: Longman. [Available from Addison-Wesley, 1 Jacob Way, Reading, MA 01867, Telephone: (800)447-2226.]

Reed, Jean. 1990. *Résumés That Get Jobs.* New York: Prentice Hall. Information on résumés, classified ads, cover letters, and interviews.

Rusch, F. R. (ed.). 1990. *Supported Employment: Models, Methods, and Issues.* Sycamore, IL: Sycamore. [Available from Sycamore Publishing Company, P.O. Box 133, Sycamore, IL 60178, Telephone: (815)756-5388.]

Sowers, J., and Powers, L. 1991. *Vocational Preparation and Employment of Students With Physical and Multiple Disabilities.* Baltimore, MD: Paul H. Brookes.

Supported Employment Parent Training Technical Assistance (SEPT/TA) Project. 1990. A reference manual for parent training about supported employment (rev. ed.). Minneapolis, MN: Pacer Center. [Available from Pacer Center, 4826 Chicago Avenue South, Minneapolis, MN 55417-1055, Telephone: (612)827-2966.]

TASH, Assessing and Teaching Job-Related Social Skills. 1990. 11201 Greenwood Avenue North, Seattle, WA 98133, (206)361-8870.

Yate, Martin John. 1988. *Résumés That Knock 'Em Dead.* Boston: Bob Adams, Inc. Includes actual résumés and explains how to put a résumé together.

— ORGANIZATIONS —

Fedcap Rehabilitation Services, Inc. 211 West 14th Street New York, NY 10011, (212)727-4200. Vocational rehabilitation and job placement services.

Foundation on Employment and Disability. 3820 Del Amo Blvd., #201, Torrance, CA 90503, (213)214-3430.

National Center on Employment for the Deaf/National Technical Institute for the Deaf. One Lomb Memorial Drive, Building 60, Rochester, NY 14623, (716)475-6834.

National Clearinghouse of Rehabilitation Training Materials. Oklahoma State University, 115 Old USDA Building, Stillwater, OK 74078, (800)223-5219. Offers reference materials.

President's Committee's Job Accommodation Network (JAN). West Virginia University, 918 Chestnut Ridge Road, Suite 1, P.O. Box 6080, Morgantown, WV 26506-6080, (800)526-7234 (Voice/TT, toll-free in U.S.); (800)526-2262 (Voice/TT, toll-free in Canada). Publications available in Spanish.

Rehabilitation Services Administration. 330 C Street, SW, Washington, DC 20202, (202)732-1362. Information, law/legislation resources.

4

LIVING ARRANGEMENTS

This chapter covers the following topics:

➤ Resources to consider in beginning your search

➤ Centers for independent living

➤ Variety of residential services available

➤ What to look for in selecting a residential facility

➤ Housing subsidies

➤ Making your residence accessible

➤ Respite care

There may be times after a student with disabilities leaves secondary education when parents will have to explore housing alternatives other than the family home. A variety of motivations for this decision may include the following:

➤ The physical, medical, economic, and psychological resources of some families to care for the needs of a family member with disabilities may diminish over time.

➤ The need to foster independence and autonomy may dictate the desirability of separate housing.

Parents who are confronted with the need for residential options may face a confusing and sometimes overwhelming fund of information. A large part of this confusion is attributable to the variety of terms used to describe these available programs, for example, *group homes* or *community residences*. In this chapter we will try to reduce the confusion caused by the different labels. In trying to unravel the many options, it is important to be as open as possible, as two group homes may be vastly different because they serve people with different levels of disability.

Three major factors will influence the types of service available to persons with disabilities.

➤ First, some residential services are available only to those who are eligible for medical assistance and county mental retardation services.

➤ Second, service options are based on the level of care needed. The family subsidy program aids families in keeping children with disabilities at home rather than placing them in a residential facility. For those who need some supervision and training to live independently but do not need care 24 hours a day, Semi-Independent Living Services (SILLS) may be an option. Community-based waivered services or placement in an intermediate care facility (group home) are options for persons who need 24-hour supervision.

➤ The third factor influencing the type of residential services available is the funding level for the programs. Unfortunately, the need for residential facilities far outweighs the availability of these resources. Some of this is due to a lack of funding, but there has also been tremendous resistance on the part of local communities to have such residences in their midst (not in my backyard). Historically, costly and lengthy legal fights have addressed this issue.

Therefore, those working with the student with disabilities must begin addressing these issues years before this need arises. Some parents report waiting five to six, or more, years for a space to open up at a facility. One of the pathways, in addition to putting their names on a list is to get parents and their children involved in the activities of a local service provider. This will enable the family to develop an ongoing relationship with that service provider, which will be helpful when space in a facility becomes available. When you begin your search for residential options, your goal should be to identify as many as possible. Knowing where to look will enable you to find contacts who can answer your questions.

RESOURCES TO CONSIDER IN BEGINNING YOUR SEARCH

Every state has numerous public agencies that are responsible for meeting the various needs of people with disabilities and their families. The names of these agencies will vary from state to state, and those involved may have to investigate or cross-reference using available agencies that assist with residential resources. Start your search with the following sources of information:

➤ Local school district's director of special education services

➤ Internet

➤ Public and university libraries

➤ Special education departments at universities

➤ ARC—The Association for Retarded Citizens (State and local chapters are usually listed in your local phone directory.)

➤ Other families or individuals who may have similar experiences

➤ Child advocacy services

CENTERS FOR INDEPENDENT LIVING (CIL)

Another important source for information and assistance is centers for independent living. These centers offer programs of services for individuals with significant disabilities, or groups of individuals with significant disabilities, that promote independence, productivity, and quality of life. The centers are run by people with disabilities who themselves have been successful in establishing independent lives. These people have both the training and personal experience to know exactly what is needed to live independently, and they have a deep commitment to assist other people with disabilities in becoming more independent.

These centers are community, consumer controlled, noninstitutional organizations. They generally offer services free of charge. There are approximately 250 CILs nationally, with at least one located in every state.

Funded by the Rehabilitation Services Administration (RSA), CILs offer a varied combination of independent living services such as:

➤   referral services
➤   independent living skills training
➤   peer counseling
➤   individual advocacy
➤   counseling services
➤   services related to securing housing or shelter
➤   rehabilitation technology
➤   mobility training
➤   life skills training
➤   interpreter and reader services
➤   personnel assistance services
➤   consumer information programs
➤   transportation assistance
➤   physical rehabilitation
➤   therapeutic treatment
➤   prostheses
➤   individual and group recreational services
➤   self-employment skills
➤   advocacy skills
➤   career options
➤   services to children
➤   preventive services
➤   community awareness programs

RESIDENTIAL MODELS

Residential Services

A residential program offers housing other than the individual's natural home, and it is usually designed for persons with similar needs in terms of age, independence, or abilities. A residential program usually provides

➤ a homelike environment with supervision and guidance as needed

➤ living experiences appropriate to the functioning level and learning needs of the individual

➤ a location within the mainstream of community life

➤ access to necessary supportive habilitative programs.

The goal of residential programs is to provide access to the highest possible quality of services that a person with certain disabilities needs, while at the same time permitting and encouraging the person to be as independent as possible.

Adult Foster Care

Adult foster care homes are provided by families who for altruistic, religious, or monetary reasons provide a home care environment for the adult with disabilities. In this residential option, the foster care family receives government reimbursement for this service. While this living arrangement is meant to be a permanent situation, no guarantees exist.

Boarding Homes

A boarding home is a residential facility that provides minimal structure and training for the adult with disabilities. These homes may provide sleeping and meal arrangements, and deal with a varied clientele with a variety of disabilities.

Family Subsidy Program

This program provides financial assistance to families to enable them to care for their children with disabilities up to age 22 at home. The Department of Human Services pays eligible families a monthly allowance for certain home care costs such as medical equipment, respite care, transportation, and special diets. Eligibility for the program is based on the needs of the family and their ability to provide the necessary level of care in the home. The program is not based on financial need.

Free-Standing Weekend Respite

This is a community-based program for families in need of respite on a planned or emergency basis. The overall objective is to afford families a reprieve from the day-to-day caregiving responsibilities. Respite provides room and board, 24-hour supervision, and appropriate recreational activities to individuals with developmental disabilities.

Group Homes

The general characteristics of group homes include

➤ a home with fewer than sixteen people

➤ a familylike structure

➤ similarity to surrounding homes in the community

➤ performance of tasks by the residents of the home to the extent of their abilities, that is, cooking, mowing the lawn, laundry, and so on.

➢ the expectation that the disabled individual will graduate to a more independent situation that will meet his or her needs and preferences

The term *group home* has taken on many meanings. The concept has certain general characteristics, but these may vary from facility to facility. Specifically, group homes are divided into two arrangements: semi-independent living arrangements and supervised living arrangements. These options differ in the following ways:

➢ staffing arrangements

➢ level of disability

➢ the need for supervision

Semi-Independent Living Arrangements (SIL)

These services provide intensive support and training to persons with disabilities 18 years of age and over to enable them to learn to live independently in the community or to maintain semi-independence. Persons eligible for SILS do not require daily support services, but are unable to live independently without some training or occasional support. SILS recipients live in their own homes or apartments, in rooming houses, or in foster homes. They often share living arrangements with other persons who have disabilities. The key characteristic is that the staff does not live in the facility. In some cases, they may be on call in cases of emergency.

Home Care Attendants or Personal Assistant Services. These auxiliary services are available to assist consumers in housekeeping and personal care needs; they enable the consumer to live more independently. They may be paid for by the individual or by public funds through Medicaid.

Supervised Living Arrangements

These services provide intensive support and training for persons with severe disabilities. Unlike semi-independent living arrangements, these facilities have full-time residential staff. This type of arrangement is usually provided for individuals who are not able to care for themselves and need full-time supervision.

Intermediate Care Facility (ICF/MR)

ICF/MR facilities are specially licensed residential settings for persons who require 24-hour care and supervision and are supported by Medicaid funds. Group homes may range in size from small six-person homes to larger institutions. Most of them are small residences, serving under sixteen people. The ICF provides a full array of direct-care and clinical services within the program model. Clinical services include psychology, social work, speech therapy, nursing, nutrition, pharmacology, and medical services. ICF admission requires that participants be Medicaid-eligible, have an IQ below 59, and manifest deficits in basic skills such as grooming and hygiene.

Supportive Living Units (SLU)

SLUs are state-funded small residential sites, typically housing one to three high-functioning individuals. These individuals may or may not be Medicaid-eligible, are typically competitively employed, and require 21 hours or less per week individual protection by a direct-care person.

Waivered Services

The term *waivered services* applies to persons with mental retardation who are currently in ICF/MRs, or who are at risk of being placed in ICF/MRs unless the waivered services can be provided to them in a home or community setting. The possible living arrangements are intended to be much less restrictive and isolated from the mainstream world than the traditional ICF/MR settings. The home or community-based residence could include a person's own parental home, a foster home, an apartment, or a small group home. These services are available to individuals who would otherwise qualify for Medicaid only if they were in an out-of-home setting.

HOW TO EVALUATE RESIDENTIAL PROGRAMS

There is no substitute for firsthand observation. When you have organized your list of potential residential programs, make appointments to visit each one. Do not hesitate to ask the following questions:

➤   What are the entry requirements?

➤   How many people live at the particular residence?

➤   Is there a waiting list?

➤   How long is the waiting list?

➤   What is the staffing pattern?

➤   What other services are provided at this residence?

➤   What are the expectations for activities outside the residence?
   –   Can the resident go to a day program?
   –   Can the resident have a part-time or weekend job?

➤   What will the costs be for the specific services provided by this residence?

➤   How is the personal money of the resident monitored?

➤   Are family visits encouraged?

➤   What kinds of household chores will the resident be responsible for?

➤   Are leisure activities part of the resident's program?

MAKING A RESIDENCE ACCESSIBLE

Whether one is building an accessible home or modifying an existing residence, the cost can be prohibitive. A home equity or other bank loan may be one financing alternative. Depending upon one's circumstances and the nature of the disability, assistance may also be obtained through medical insurance, medical and social services, income support, or vocational services from any of a number of different resources. Consumer-oriented disability organizations and rehabilitation facilities may also provide information resources on funding assistance available in the local community.

HOUSING SUBSIDIES

Section 8 Housing

Section 8 refers to rent subsidy payments by the government to allow an individual to secure decent, safe, and sanitary housing in private accommodations. The income limitations for eligibility are determined by information from the local housing authorities. This program comes under the U.S. Department of Housing and Urban Development (HUD).

The specific steps required in applying for rental assistance are:

1. An application must be completed and filed with the local housing authority.

2. Eligibility is then determined, based on the intended type of occupancy (elderly or disabled) and income.

3. It is up to the parent or the young person to find suitable housing on the open market.

4. This housing must be inspected by the local housing authority and meet demanding quality standards.

5. Once the housing has passed inspection, it must be determined if the landlord is interested in participating in Section 8 housing.

6. If it is determined that rent and utilities do not exceed the fair market rent, and the landlord is in agreement, the housing may be leased.

Section 202 Housing

Section 202 refers to a program that provides direct loans for the construction of housing for three specific populations:

➢ individuals with developmental disabilities

➢ those with chronic mental illness

➢ those with physical disabilities

These funds are intended for the construction of group facilities for the disabled. You can get further information on this subsidy from your local housing authority.

RESPITE CARE

What Is Respite Care?

Respite care refers to short-term, temporary care provided to people with disabilities in order that their families can take a break from the daily routine of caregiving. Respite care services may sometimes involve overnight care for an extended period of time.

One of the important purposes of respite care is to give family members time and temporarily relieve the stress they may experience while providing extra care for a son or daughter with mental retardation or other disability. Respite care enables families to take vacations, or just a few hours of time off. Respite care is often referred to as "a gift of time."

Periodic respite care can help a parent relax for a while and come back revitalized and better able to care for a son or daughter. Respite care not only provides caregivers a break but also gives the child a change in his or her daily routine.

Who Provides Respite Services?

Most programs are managed by affiliates or chapters of national organizations such as ARC, Easter Seal Society, and United Cerebral Palsy Associations in cooperation with local hotels (US/GAO). Many other programs are provided by such local organizations as churches, schools, and other nonprofit groups.

What Kinds of Services Are Provided?

Services are provided in many ways, depending on the provider, the needs of the family, and available funds. Some respite programs send a caregiver to the family's home. Others require that the individual come to a day care center or respite group home.

In some programs, the care is provided by a host family that also has a family member with a disability. They usually provide respite services in exchange for the same services from another family. These programs are called *host family* or *exchange* programs.

Emergency respite services are also important. Parents must be able to access services on short notice in the event that a family emergency occurs.

Are There Eligibility Requirements for Respite Services?

In almost all state-funded programs, eligibility is based on the child's age and disabilities. Family income is also usually considered.

Some questions to ask about a respite care program are:

➢ How are care providers screened?

➢ What is the training and level of experience of the care providers?

➢ Will care providers need additional training to meet specific family needs?

➢ How, and by whom, are the care providers supervised?

➢ What happens during the time the children are receiving services? Are there organized activities? How are meals handled?

➢ Does the program maintain current information about each child's medical and other needs? Is there a written care plan?

➢ What procedures does the program have for emergencies?

➢ Can parents meet and interview the people who care for the children?

➢ How far ahead of time do parents need to call to arrange for services?

➢ Are families limited to a certain number of hours of services?

➢ Does the program provide transportation?

➢ Can the provider take care of brothers and sisters as well?

➢ What is the cost of services? How is payment arranged? (Karp n.d.)

A FINAL WORD

Just as in the school setting where the policy fosters the least restrictive educational environment, it follows that the same philosophy should be encouraged in seeking out adult living arrangements. This least restrictive independent arrangement may require utilization of many agencies, support personnel, family, and so on. Everything should be done to attain an individual's personal least restrictive living arrangement.

Further, individuals with disabilities should be aware that funding may be available to assist in making a residence adaptive to personal needs—ramps, modifications in doorways, or bathrooms. Explore this option with your local center for independent living.

— GLOSSARY —

Client Assistance Project—a federally mandated program to advocate for applicants and consumers. CAP helps consumers to understand Department of Rehabilitation requirements and services, resolves communication problems, informs consumers of their rights and responsibilities, and represents consumers at administrative reviews and hearings.

habilitative programs—programs that provide an educational approach, used with exceptional children, that is directed toward the development of the necessary skills required for successful adulthood.

intentional communities—residential option in which people with disabilities and without disabilities choose to live together. The arrangements vary from community to community. L'Arche homes and Camp Hill villages are examples of intentional communities.

local service provider—a not-for-profit organization, which may or may not be part of a national organization, that provides information and services to people with disabilities.

natural home—a residential option in which people continue to live with their natural families or with other relatives.

— REFERENCES —

Carney, I.; Getzel, E. E.; and Uhl, M. 1992. *Developing Respite Care Services in Your Community: A Planning Guide.* Richmond, VA: The Respite Resource Project, Virginia Institute for Developmental Disabilities. [Available from the Respite Resource Project, Virginia Institute for Developmental Disabilities, Virginia Commonwealth University, P.O. Box 843020, Richmond, VA 23284-3020. Telephone: (804)828-8587.]

Garee, B. (ed.). 1996. *An Accessible Home of Your Own* Accent Books and Products Pub., P.O. Box 700, Bloomington, IL 61702 (800)787-8444.

Garee, B. (ed.). 1996. *A Place to Live.* Accent Books Pub., P.O. Box 700, Bloomington, IL 61702 (800)787-8444.

Hill, J. W., and Ledman, S. M. 1990. *Integrated After-School Day Care: A Solution for Respite Care Needs in Your Community.* Richmond, VA: Virginia Institute for Developmental Disabilities, Virginia Commonwealth University, Respite Resource Project.

Janicki, M. P.; Krauss, M. W.; and Seltzer, M. M. 1988. *Community Residences for Persons With Developmental Disabilities: Here to Stay.* Baltimore, MD: Paul H. Brookes.

Karp, N., and Ellis, G. J. (eds.). 1992. *Time Out for Families: Epilepsy and Respite Care.* Landover, MD: Epilepsy Foundation of America. [Available from the Epilepsy Foundation of America. Telephone: (800)213-5821.]

Karp, Naomi, et al. n.d. *Respite Care: A Guide for Parents.* Washington, DC: CSR, Incorporated and Association for the Care of Children's Health.

Kniest, B. A., and Garland, C. W. 1991. *Partners: A Manual for Family-Centered Respite Care.* Lightfoot, VA: Child Development Resources; Richmond, VA: Virginia Institute for Developmental Disabilities, Virginia Commonwealth University, Respite Resource Project.

Racino, J. A.; Walker, P.; O'Conner, S.; and Taylor, S. J. 1993. *Housing, Support and Community: Choices in Strategy for Adults With Disabilities.* Baltimore MD: Paul H. Brookes.

Respite Care: An Overview of Federal, Selected State, and Private Programs. Report number GAO 90-125 (September 1990). Washington, DC: United States General Accounting Office, (US/GAO).

— ORGANIZATIONS —

Adaptive Environments Center. 374 Congress Street, Suite 301, Boston, MA 02110. (617)695-1225 (V/TT). (617)482-8099 (fax). The Adaptive Environments Center, a non-profit organization, offers consultation, workshops, courses, conferences, and resource materials on accessible and adaptive design and accessibility legislation, standards, and guidelines. The library is open to the public.

ARCH National Resource Center. 1995. *ARCH National Directory of Crisis Nurseries and Respite Care Programs.* Chapel Hill, NC. [Available from ARCH National Resource Center, Chapel Hill Training-Outreach Project, 800 Eastowne Drive, Suite 105, Chapel Hill, NC 27514. Telephone: (800)473-1727; (919)490-5577.]

Barrier Free Environments (BFE). P.O. Box 30634, Water Garden, Highway 70 West, Raleigh, NC 27622, (919)782-7823 (V/TT). Barrier Free Environments (BFE) is a design firm specializing exclusively in the design of products and buildings to be used by aging people and people with disabilities.

Center for Accessible Housing. North Carolina State University, Box 8613, Raleigh, NC 27695-8613, (919)515-3082 (V/TT). The Center for Accessible Housing was established in 1989 by the National Institute on Disability and Rehabilitation Research (NIDRR) to improve the quality and availability of housing for people with disabilities. The center provides assistance and information to individuals and industry through research, collaborative efforts with manufacturers, training, and information services.

Housing for Elderly and Handicapped People Division. 451 7th Street SW, Room 6116, Washington, DC 20410, (202)708-2866. The Housing for Elderly and Handicapped People Division administers the Section 811 Program—Supportive Housing for Persons With Disabilities. This program provides capital advances to private, nonprofit organizations for the development of housing with supportive services for people who have physical or developmental disabilities or who are chronically mentally ill.

JARC-Jewish Association for Residential Care. 28366 Franklin Road, Southfield, MI 48034, (810)352-5272. Provides residential care and support services.

Developmental Disability Councils. 200 Independence Avenue SW, Washington, DC 20201, (202)245-2890. Councils in each state provide training and technical assistance to local and state agencies.

National Council on Independent Living. 4th Street and Broadway, Troy, NY 12180, (518)274-1979. Information, referrals, and advocacy services.

National Handicap Housing Institute, Inc. (NHHI). 4556 Lake Drive, Robbinsdale, MN 55422, (612)535-9771. The NHHI was incorporated in 1975 as a tax-exempt charitable organization providing services related to the development of barrier-free housing for young adults with physical disabilities.

5

TRANSPORTATION CONCERNS

This chapter covers the following topics:

➤ Rights to public access

➤ Federal legislation that supports travel training

➤ What is travel training

➤ What happens during travel training

➤ Skills required for traveling independently

➤ When should young people with disabilities enter a travel training program?

➤ Why are travel training programs necessary?

➤ Who should provide travel training?

➤ Paratransit systems

➤ Print resources available

➤ Organizations available to answer travel training concerns

Today, the lack of access to transportation that many individuals with disabilities have experienced is changing. The Americans With Disabilities Act (ADA) recognizes the critical role that public transportation plays in the lives of many people and mandates that public transportation systems, where available, become accessible to people with disabilities. Unfortunately, availability of transportation is not the only impediment to independent travel for people with disabilities. For many individuals, learning how to travel on public transportation requires systematic training. Travel training, then, is often a crucial element in empowering people with disabilities to use the newly accessible transportation systems in our country.

Transportation provides us all with access to the wider opportunities of employment, postsecondary education, job training programs, and recreation, to name a few. Traveling by car, by cab, or by such public transportation systems as bus or subway enables us to go to work and come home, go to school or other training programs, visit friends, take care of daily needs like grocery shopping, and enjoy recreational activities. Many individuals with disabilities have traditionally been isolated from these societal opportunities, because they lacked a means of transportation. For many, driving a car was not possible, due to a visual, physical, or cognitive disability. Public transportation systems were often inaccessible due to structural barriers. Still other individuals were unable to use the transportation systems that were available, because they lacked the training, or know-how, to use these systems safely.

WHAT IS TRAVEL TRAINING?

Travel training is short-term, comprehensive, intensive instruction designed to teach students with disabilities how to travel safely and independently on public transportation. The goal of travel training is to train students to travel independently to a regularly visited destination and back. Specially trained personnel provide the travel training on a one-to-one basis. Students learn travel skills while following a particular route, generally to school or a worksite, and are taught the safest, most direct route. The travel trainer is responsible for making sure the student experiences and understands the realities of public transportation and learns the skills required for safe and independent travel.

The term *travel training* is often used generically to refer to a program that provides instruction in travel skills to individuals with any disability except visual impairment. Individuals who have a visual impairment receive travel training from orientation and mobility specialists usually under the jurisdiction of a state commission for the blind. Travel trainers have the task of understanding how different disabilities affect a person's ability to travel independently, and devising customized strategies to teach travel skills that address the specific needs of people with those disabilities.

A travel trainer usually begins training a student at the student's residence, which allows the trainer to

- ➤ observe the student in a familiar environment
- ➤ reassure the family through daily contact
- ➤ assess the student's home environment at regular travel times for potential problems

In a quality travel training program, a travel trainer works with one student at a time. The trainer follows the travel route with the student and instructs the student in dealing with such problems as getting lost or taking a detour around a construction site. The trainer should teach the student to make decisions, deal with the consequences of decisions, and maintain appropriate safety and behavior standards.

When to Enter a Travel Training Program

Most people enter travel training between the ages of 15 and 21; however, it may be appropriate for some children to be introduced to travel training at an earlier age.

FEDERAL LEGISLATION SUPPORTING THE PROVISION OF TRAVEL TRAINING

For many students transportation is critical to transition, since transportation affects how people live, work, play, and participate in their community. Parents and professionals must advocate for the inclusion of travel training in the Individualized Education

Program (IEP). Access to transportation, and the ability to use it, can open doors and provide a means to many otherwise unavailable opportunities for persons with disabilities.

Together, ADA (Americans With Disabilities Act) and IDEA (Individuals With Disabilities Education Act) provide individuals with disabilities, their families, school systems, service providers, community agencies, and transit systems with compelling incentives to work together to ensure that students learn how to use accessible transportation.

Providing students with travel training can reduce expenses for school districts, local governments, transit providers, agencies, or any organization that provides transportation. The cost of using public transportation is significantly less than the cost of using a contracted private car or private bus service. While the cost of training a student can be substantial, in the long run that cost is a worthwhile investment, since the student will gain independence and henceforth will assume responsibility for the cost of using public transportation.

THE IMPORTANCE OF TRAVEL TRAINING

Being able to get around on one's own is an important component of independence; this is as true for people with disabilities as it is for those without disabilities. Nearly all people who have disabilities can (with training and the use of accessible vehicles) board, travel on, and exit a public transportation vehicle. A certified travel training program is often needed, however, to teach people who have a disability to do these procedures safely and independently. Programs that maintain high-quality procedures for travel training are crucial in helping people who have a disability to develop autonomy and practice their right to move freely through a community.

WHO PROVIDES TRAVEL TRAINING?

A logical place to implement travel training programs is within the public school system. As the primary providers of education for students with a disability, local school districts have a full range of resources available to develop quality travel training programs. Since students are part of a school system for many consecutive years, educators can plan and deliver a full program of travel instruction. Then, as students become young adults and are close to exiting the school system, explicit travel training can become part of their education and can form the basis of the transition from school transportation to public transportation. While the public school system is the optimal environment in which to begin travel training, individuals with disabilities can also get travel training from independent living centers or similar agencies.

Society, too, benefits when people with disabilities participate actively in everyday life. Travel training programs can enable students with disabilities to become adults who can travel to and from their jobs without support, who are involved citizens of their communities, and who have the opportunity to live independently.

PARATRANSIT SYSTEMS

Paratransit service is a shared ride service (van or sedan) in compliance with the Complementary Paratransit Service provisions of the Americans With Disabilities Act of 1990 (ADA).

While the specific provisions of paratransit systems vary from locality to locality, paratransit usually provides door-to-door transportation for persons with disabilities or mobility impairments who are unable to use public buses. *Door-to-door* usually means transportation to and from the main entrance of the place of destination. It is the responsibility of the individual to be ready and waiting at the main entrance for pickup.

A FINAL WORD

While many transportation options for the disabled exist in certain areas, there is still work to be done in making all public transportation accessible. The availability of these options must be coordinated with the skills required to use such services. These skills begin early in one's life and must be reinforced continuously if one is to move toward a world of independence.

— GLOSSARY —

FTA—Federal Transportation Administration.

IDEA—The Education of the Handicapped Act, Public Law (P.L.) 94-142, was passed by Congress in 1975 and amended by P.L. 99-457 in 1986 to ensure that all children with disabilities would have a free, appropriate public education available to them that would meet their unique needs. It was again amended in 1990, and the name was changed to IDEA (Individuals With Disabilities Act).

RTAP—Rapid Transit Assistance Program is a program of the Federal Transit Administration (FTA) that provides information and technical assistance on all issues related to rural and specialized transit. RTAP has both a national program and state programs that work together in partnership.

TRIS—Transportation Research Information Services is a unique on-line computerized information file that contains both abstracts of completed research and profiles of research in progress.

— REFERENCES —

Jacobsen, W. 1993. *The Art and Science of Teaching Orientation and Mobility to Persons With Visual Impairments.* New York: American Foundation for the Blind. [Available from the American Foundation for the Blind, AFB Order Dept., 11 Penn Plaza, Suite 300, New York, NY 10001 Telephone: (800)232-3044.]

Moon, S. 1994. *Making Schools and Community Recreation Fun for Everyone.* Baltimore, MD: Paul H. Brookes. [Available from Paul H. Brookes Publishing Company, P.O. Box 10624, Baltimore, MD 21285-0624. Telephone: (800)638-3775.]

Uslan, M. M.; Peck, A. F.; Wiener, W. R. and Stern, A. (eds.). 1990. *Access to Mass Transit for Blind and Visually Impaired Travelers.* New York: American Foundation for the Blind. [Available from the American Foundation for the Blind, AFB Order Dept., 11 Penn Plaza, Suite 300, New York, NY 10001. Telephone: (800)232-3044.]

Transportation Research Board (TRB). 1993. *Accessible Transportation and Mobility.* Washington, DC: TRB. [Available from Transportation Board, Box 289, Washington, DC 20055. Telephone: (202)334-3213/3214. (*Note:* This publication is technically written for an audience of transportation providers.)]

West, J. (ed.). 1996. *Implementing the Americans With Disabilities Act.* Cambridge, MA: Blackwell Publishers. [Available from Blackwell Publishers, P.O. Box 20, Williston, VT 05495-0020. Telephone: (800)216-2522.]

— ORGANIZATIONS —

ADA in Action. (800)949-4232 ADA (Americans with Disabilities Act) in Action Centers are regional centers funded by the U.S. Department of Education, National Institute on Disability and Rehabilitation Research, to provide technical assistance, materials dissemination, and training on the Americans With Disabilities Act. This 800 number will automatically connect you with the office that serves your region. Call and ask for their publications list; it has an entire section on Public Transportation.

American Foundation for the Blind. Information Center, 11 Penn Plaza, Suite 300, New York, NY 10001. Telephone: (800)232-5463. Web address: http://www.afb.org/afb. E-mail: afbinfo@afb.org. A nonprofit organization founded in 1921 and recognized as Helen Keller's cause in the United States, the American Foundation for the Blind (AFB) is a leading national resource for people who are blind or visually impaired, the organizations who serve them, and the general public. The mission of the AFB is to enable people who are blind or visually impaired to achieve equality of access and opportunity that will ensure freedom of choice in their lives.

Center for Transportation, Education, and Development. University of Wisconsin Milwaukee, 161 West Wisconsin Ave., Ste. 6000, Milwaukee, WI 53203. Telephone: (414)227-3337. The mission of the Center for Transportation, Education, and Development is to provide quality education programs to transportation professionals. The center provides noncredit continuing education that meets the needs of administrators, managers, supervisors, drivers, and consumers of transportation services. Their training sessions deal with subjects such as scheduling and dispatching, travel training, paratransit, passenger assistance, and cost containment.

Clearinghouse on School/Special Education. Sweetwood Foundation, c/o Serif Press, Inc., 1331 H Street NW, Suite 11OLL, Washington, DC 20005. Telephone: (202)737-4650. This information clearinghouse provides its members in school transportation with an information exchange service. Also available are a newsletter, *Transporting Students With Disabilities,* bibliographies of existing reports, legislation, surveys, test results, articles and video tapes, and a library of additional resources.

Community Transportation Assistance Program (CTAP). c/o Community Transition Association of America (CTAA), 1440 New York Ave. NW, Suite 440, Washington, DC 20005. Telephone: (800)527-82V9; (202)628-1480. CTAP is funded through a grant with the U.S. Department of Health and Human Services. It is a technical assistance and training project that includes a national transportation clearinghouse serving human services agencies, and provides technical assistance, electronic bulletin board services, peer-to-peer network, and training workshops and materials.

Disabled Americans for Accessible Public Transit. 12 Broadway Denver, CO 80203 (303)936-1110.

MedEscort International, Inc. ABE International Airport PO Box 8766, Allentown, PA 18105 (215)791-3111. Offers specially trained escorts for individuals with disabilities who cannot travel alone.

National Institute for Accessible Transportation. 1350 New York Avenue NW, Suite 613, Washington, DC 20005. Telephone: (800)659-6428 (Voice/TTY).

Project ACTION. Accessible Community Transportation in our Nation, funded by the Federal Transit Administration (FTA) and administered by the National Easter Seals Society, is a national research and demonstration program established to improve access to transportation services for people with disabilities and assist transit providers in implementing the Americans With Disabilities Act (ADA). Call to get a copy of Project ACTION's extensive publication and report list.

Rural Transit Assistance Program. National Resource Center, c/o Community Transportation Association of America, 1440 New York Ave. NW, Suite 440, Washington, DC 20005. Telephone: (800)527 8279; (202)628-1480. RTAP is a program of the Federal Transit Administration (FTA) that provides information and technical assistance on all issues related to rural and specialized transit. RTAP has both a national program and state programs that work together in partnership. On the national level, the National Resource Center offers training materials, technical assistance, and communications with the industry. Contact RTAP to get a list of your state's RTAP contacts.

Transportation Research Information Services (TRIS). National Research Council, 2101 Constitution Avenue NW, Washington, DC 20418. Telephone: (202)334-3250. Transportation Research Information Services (TRIS) is a unique on-line computerized information file that contains both abstracts of completed research and profiles of research in progress. The TRIS mission is to acquire, provide access to, and disseminate reference materials for all transportation research projects and publications useful to administrators, engineers, operators, researchers, and other members of the transportation community. TRIS can be accessed directly through DIALOG Information System File 63 or by contacting them directly.

US Architectural and Transportation Barriers Compliance Board. The Access Board, Suite 1000, 1331 F Street NW, Washington, DC 20004-1111. Telephone: (800)872-2253 (voice/TTY); (202)272-5434 (voice/TTY). Since 1973, the Access Board has been the only independent federal agency whose primary mission is accessibility for people with disabilities. If the board finds that a building or facility is covered by the Act and does not meet accessibility standards, it tries to resolve the complaint; if the complaint cannot be resolved, the board can take legal action to gain compliance.

University Transportation Centers Clearinghouse. Ann Marie Hutchinson, Pennsylvania State University, Research Office Building, University Park, PA 16802-4710. Telephone: (814)663-3614. The clearinghouse collects research studies and publishes an annual report on the work of the various university transportation centers. It maintains a library and can refer inquiries to sources of studies and publications, and disseminate research results.

6

RECREATIONAL AND
LEISURE OPTIONS

This chapter covers the following:

➢   The importance of leisure activities

➢   The advantages of special leisure programs designed for individuals with disabilities

➢   Leisure activity concerns of individuals with disabilities

➢   Mastering leisure skill activities

➢   A vast number of available leisure resources

When the student is involved in the transition from school to adult life, a healthy part of this journey should include leisure activities. You can discover a child's leisure interests by having him or her sample a variety of activities. Parents of very young children in today's society normally expose them to a wide variety of experiences such as

➢   dance classes

➢   Little League

➢   music lessons

➢   scouting

➢   sports activities

➢   cultural experiences

➢   travel

➢   art lessons

As the student without disabilities grows older, this process of sampling leisure interests depends less on the parents and more on the peer group. For young people with disabilities, however, parents and other family members may continue to guide or structure leisure experiences. This extended period of parental guidance and involvement should be considered a realistic part of the transitional process to adulthood for a student with disabilities. Learning specific leisure skills can be an important component for successful integration into community recreation programs. Research has shown that leisure skill training contributes to a sense of competence, social interaction, and appropriate behavior.

ADVANTAGES OF SPECIAL LEISURE PROGRAMS

One of the issues that parents and professionals have to address is whether a child should participate in activities designed specifically for people with disabilities or enter activities geared for a more mainstreamed population. The advantages of a special program designed for children with disabilities follow:

➤ may allow the only opportunity for some children with severe disabilities to participate, for example, Special Olympics

➤ allows for a sense of group identity

➤ provides a setting for social interaction

➤ creates a more level playing field so that the disabled individual's *abilities* become the focus rather than the disability

On the other hand, concentrating on "disabled only" activities may unnecessarily exclude individuals from many leisure opportunities, and prevents interaction with the nondisabled community.

INDIVIDUAL CONCERNS WHEN FACED WITH LEISURE ACTIVITIES

One of the greatest concerns of individuals with disabilities is the problems they may face assimilating into the social world. Many students receive special services while in school that expose them to other children with disabilities. This social interaction and connection provides a foundation for improving social skills. Once school experience ends and the child is confronted with the mainstream world, however, many of these social opportunities are not available and social isolation is often the result. Social isolation is probably the most painful aspect that individuals with disabilities face when they enter adulthood. Therefore, a parent, particularly, plays a crucial role in assisting the child by providing the exposure to leisure and recreational activities. Parents may often find themselves the only agents for this particular aspect of life—especially once the child leaves the school setting.

MASTERING LEISURE ACTIVITY SKILLS

Mastering a leisure activity skill provides many advantages for the individuals with disabilities. This process will

➤ increase the individual's interest level

➤ increase self-esteem and confidence through the mastery of skills

➤ provide the individual with communication topics for social interaction

➤ broaden the individual's knowledge base

As opportunities for recreation and leisure are investigated by both the parents and the child, several considerations may arise:

1. What is the experiential and sensitivity level of the people running the program in an integrated activity?

2. How much will the activity or program cost?

3. How will the individual get to the activity?

4. Is the activity integrated?

5. Does the individual need or want to have someone supervise or accompany him or her while participating in the activity?

6. Will the activity occur regularly? An optimal leisure plan would include a balance of ongoing and one-time-only activities.

AVAILABLE LEISURE ACTIVITIES

Once the leisure activities available within a community have been examined, options must be weighed and selected to ensure continuous and growing experiences. The value that individuals with disabilities attach to each of the questions above will depend on their interests, residential situation, and accessibility.

A wide variety of leisure activities is available; these activities may be either integrated or specifically geared to those with disabilities. While integrated or mainstreamed activities abound, special programs may be harder to find. As a result, we are including two lists. The first list of sources of special needs programs throughout the country is arranged by specific leisure and recreational activity. The second list includes complete names, addresses, phone numbers, and descriptions of these sources, alphabetically by state.

Sources of Specific Leisure and Recreational Activities

Activities are listed here in alphabetical order. The list is provided as a partial reference only. See the following listing of organizations by state, p. 96. Contact the specific organizations listed for other possible sources.

ADVENTURE

Challenge Alaska

AEROBICS

Sports Association, Gaylord Hospital (CT)

RIC Skiers—Wirtz Sports Program (IL)
(*See also* Fitness)

AEROBICS—AQUATIC

Eagle Mount—Great Falls (MT)

ALL-TERRAIN VEHICLES

Disabled Sports USA—Lakeside Chapter (NV)

ARCHERY

Sports Association, Gaylord Hospital (CT)

Courage Center (MN)

Courage Duluth (MN)

Variety Wheelchair Arts and Sports Assn. (TX)

BASEBALL—LITTLE LEAGUE

Challenge New Mexico

BASEBALL—GENERAL

Disabled Sports USA—Lakeside Chapter (NV)

Challenge New Mexico

BASKETBALL—GENERAL

RIC Skiers—Wirtz Sports Program (IL)

Disabled Sports USA—Lakeside Chapter (NV)

Challenge New Mexico

Deutsch Institute (PA)

Variety Wheelchair Arts and Sports Assn. (TX)

National Ability Center (UT)

BASKETBALL—WHEELCHAIR

Sports Association, Gaylord Hospital (CT)

RIC Skiers—Wirtz Sports Program (IL)

Wheelchair Sports and Recreation (MA)

Courage Duluth (MN)

Three Rivers Adaptive Sports (TRAS) (PA)

Amputee Connection Inc., dba Just a Little Inconvenience (TX)

Disabled Sports Association of North Texas (TX)

BIKING

(*See* Cycling)

BILLIARDS—WHEELCHAIR

Deutsch Institute (PA)

BOCCE

Mesa Association of Sports for the Disabled (AZ)

Deutsch Institute (PA)

Disabled Sports Association of North Texas (TX)

BOWLING

Mesa Association of Sports for the Disabled (AZ)

Disabled Sports USA—Lakeside Chapter (NV)

Deutsch Institute (PA)

Three Rivers Adaptive Sports (TRAS) (PA)

Disabled Sports Association of North Texas (TX)

Variety Wheelchair Arts and Sports Assn. (TX)

Richmond Athletes With Disabilities (RAD) Sports (VA)

Bowls—Lawn

Disabled Sports USA—Lakeside Chapter (NV)

Camping—Backpacking

Breckenridge Outdoor Education Center (CO)
(*See also* Wilderness Experiences)

Camping—Cabin

Challenge Alaska
(*See also* Wilderness Experiences)

Camping—General

Challenge Alaska

Challenge Alaska, Kenai Peninsula

Challenge Alaska Southeast

California Handicapped Skiers

Disabled Sports USA of Northern California

The Unrecables (Los Angeles Chapter of Disabled Sports USA)

Breckenridge Outdoor Education Center (CO)

National Sports Center for the Disabled (CO)

Baltimore Adapted Recreation and Sports (BARS) (MD)

Eagle Mount—Great Falls (MT)

Three Rivers Adaptive Sports (TRAS) (PA)

Variety Wheelchair Arts and Sports Assn. (TX)

National Ability Center (UT)

Options for Independence (UT)

Vermont Adaptive Ski and Sports Association

Disabled Sports USA Northwest ("Team USAble") (WA)
(*See also* Wilderness Experiences)

Camps—Summer

Alpine Alternatives (AK)
(*See also* Wilderness Experiences)

Canoeing

Alpine Alternatives (AK)

Challenge Alaska

Challenge Alaska Southeast

California Handicapped Skiers

Disabled Sports USA of Northern California

Breckenridge Outdoor Education Center (CO)

Maine Access-able Adventures

Baltimore Adapted Recreation and Sports (BARS) (MD)

Wheelchair Sports and Recreation (MA)

Cannonsburg Challenged Ski Association (MI)

Disabled Sports USA—Lakeside Chapter (NV)

New England Handicapped Sports (NH)

Three Rivers Adaptive Sports (TRAS) (PA)

Variety Wheelchair Arts and Sports Assn. (TX)

Options for Independence (UT)

Vermont Adaptive Ski and Sports Association

Richmond Athletes With Disabilities (RAD) Sports (VA)

Disabled Sports USA Northwest ("Team USAble") (WA)

CLIMBING—ROCK

Challenge Alaska

Adaptive Sports Center of Crested Butte (CO)

Breckenridge Outdoor Education Center (CO)

National Sports Center for the Disabled (CO)

Maine Access-able Adventures

Disabled Sports USA—Lakeside Chapter (NV)

CONDITIONING

(*See* Strength and Conditioning)

CULTURAL ACTIVITIES

Challenge Alaska

CYCLING—GENERAL

Challenge Alaska Southeast

Adaptive Sports Center of Crested Butte (CO)

National Sports Center for the Disabled (CO)

Maine Access-able Adventures

Baltimore Adapted Recreation and Sports (BARS) (MD)

Wheelchair Sports and Recreation (MA)

Disabled Sports USA—Lakeside Chapter (NV)

Northeast Passage (NH)

Three Trackers of Ohio

Three Rivers Adaptive Sports (TRAS) (PA)

Variety Wheelchair Arts and Sports Assn. (TX)

Vermont Adaptive Ski and Sports Association

CYCLING—HAND

National Sports Center for the Disabled (CO)

Baltimore Adapted Recreation and Sports (BARS) (MD)

Wheelchair Sports and Recreation (MA)

    Northeast Passage (NH)

    Three Rivers Adaptive Sports (TRAS) (PA)

    Vermont Adaptive Ski and Sports Association

CYCLING—MOUNTAIN

    Adaptive Sports Center of Crested Butte (CO)

    National Sports Center for the Disabled (CO)

EQUESTRIAN

    Alpine Alternatives (AK)

    Adaptive Sports Center of Crested Butte (CO)

    Maine Access-able Adventures

    Eagle Mount—Great Falls (MT)

    I Am Third Foundation—dba Eagle Mount (MT)

    Disabled Sports USA—Lakeside Chapter (NV)

    Challenge New Mexico

    Variety Wheelchair Arts and Sports Assn. (TX)

    National Ability Center (UT)

    Vermont Adaptive Ski and Sports Association

FENCING

    RIC Skiers—Wirtz Sports Program (IL)

    Variety Wheelchair Arts and Sports Assn. (TX)

FIELD AND TRACK

    (*See* Track and Field)

FISHING—DEEP SEA

    Challenge Alaska

FISHING—GENERAL

    Challenge Alaska

    Challenge Alaska, Kenai Peninsula

    Challenge Alaska Southeast

    California Handicapped Skiers

    National Sports Center for the Disabled (CO)

    Wheelchair Sports and Recreation (MA)

    Disabled Sports USA—Lakeside Chapter (NV)

    Paraplegics on Independent Nature Trips (POINT) (TX)

    Variety Wheelchair Arts and Sports Assn. (TX)

    National Ability Center (UT)

    Vermont Adaptive Ski and Sports Association

    Richmond Athletes With Disabilities (RAD) Sports (VA)

FITNESS

   Challenge Alaska

   Sports Association, Gaylord Hospital (CT)

   Wheelchair Sports and Recreation (MA)

   Disabled Sports USA—Lakeside Chapter (NV)

   A.S.P.I.R.E. (Upstate New York)

   Variety Wheelchair Arts and Sports Assn. (TX)

   Richmond Athletes With Disabilities (RAD) Sports (VA)
     (*See also* Aerobics)

FOOTBALL

   Disabled Sports USA—Lakeside Chapter (NV)

   Variety Wheelchair Arts and Sports Assn. (TX)

GARDENING

   (*See* Horticulture and Gardening)

GOLF—AQUATIC

   I Am Third Foundation—dba Eagle Mount (MT)

GOLF—MINIATURE

   National Sports Center for the Disabled (CO)

GOLF—STANDARD

   Challenge Alaska

   California Handicapped Skiers

   Colorado Discover Ability

   Golf 4 Fun (CO)

   National Sports Center for the Disabled (CO)

   Sports Association, Gaylord Hospital (CT)

   RIC Skiers—Wirtz Sports Program (IL)

   I Am Third Foundation—dba Eagle Mount—Billings (MT)

   New England Handicapped Sports (NH)

   Waterville Valley Foundation (NH)

   Disabled Ski Program at Ski Windham (NY)

   Three Trackers of Ohio

   National Ability Center (UT)

   Richmond Athletes With Disabilities (RAD) Sports (VA)

GYMNASTICS

   Disabled Sports USA—Lakeside Chapter (NV)

HIKING AND NATURE WALKS

   Alpine Alternatives (AK)

National Sports Center for the Disabled (CO)

Baltimore Adapted Recreation and Sports (BARS) (MD)

Eagle Mount—Great Falls (MT)

Disabled Sports USA—Lakeside Chapter (NV)

National Ability Center (UT)

Options for Independence (UT)
  (*See also* Wilderness Experiences)

HOCKEY—ICE

Challenge Alaska

Vermont Adaptive Ski and Sports Association

HOCKEY—SLED

Northeast Passage (NH)

HOCKEY—SLEDGE

Wheelchair Sports and Recreation (MA)

Vermont Adaptive Ski and Sports Association

HOCKEY—WHEELCHAIR

U.S. Electric Wheelchair Hockey Association (MN)

HORSE

(*See* Equestrian)

HORTICULTURE AND GARDENING

I Am Third Foundation—dba Eagle Mount (MT)

Disabled Sports USA—Lakeside Chapter (NV)

HUNTING

Alabama Handicapped Sportsmen

Wheelchair Sports and Recreation (MA)

I Am Third Foundation—dba Eagle Mount-Billings (MT)

KAYAKING

Challenge Alaska

Challenge Alaska Southeast

California Handicapped Skiers

Disabled Sports USA of Northern California

The Unrecables (Los Angeles Chapter of Disabled Sports USA)

Maine Access-able Adventures

Baltimore Adapted Recreation and Sports (BARS) (MD)

Wheelchair Sports and Recreation (MA)

Northeast Passage (NH)

Three Rivers Adaptive Sports (TRAS) (PA)
Variety Wheelchair Arts and Sports Assn. (TX)
Disabled Sports USA Northwest ("Team USAble") (WA)

LEISURE
(*See* Social and Leisure)

MARTIAL ARTS
Wheelchair Sports and Recreation (MA)
Disabled Sports USA—Lakeside Chapter (NV)
Northeast Passage (NH)
Variety Wheelchair Arts and Sports Assn. (TX)
Richmond Athletes With Disabilities (RAD) Sports (VA)

MASSAGE
Northeast Passage (NH)

MOUNTAINEERING
(*See* Climbing—Rock)

NATURE
(*See* Hiking and Nature Walks, Wilderness Experiences)

OUTREACH (AMPUTEE AND SPINAL CORD ON CALL)
A.S.P. I.R.E. (Upstate New York)

PADDLE SPORTS
(*See* Canoeing, Kayaking)

PERSONAL IMPROVEMENT
Breckenridge Outdoor Education Center (CO)
A.S.P. I.R.E. (New York/Long Island)

PERSONAL WATER CRAFT
California Handicapped Skiers

PING-PONG
(*See* Tennis—Table)

POLO—WATER
Disabled Sports USA—Lakeside Chapter (NV)

POWERLIFTING AND WEIGHTLIFTING
RIC Skiers—Wirtz Sports Program (IL)
Wheelchair Sports and Recreation (MA)
Disabled Sports USA—Lakeside Chapter (NV)
Warriors on Wheels (NY)

Variety Wheelchair Arts and Sports Assn. (TX)

National Ability Center (UT)

RACQUETBALL

Baltimore Adapted Recreation and Sports (BARS) (MD)

Wheelchair Sports and Recreation (MA)

Disabled Sports USA—Lakeside Chapter (NV)

Northeast Passage (NH)

REHAB—MISC.

Physically Adapted Recreation and Sports (FL)

RIC Skiers—Wirtz Sports Program (IL)

Amputees Coming Together of East Tennessee

RIVER RAFTING

Challenge Alaska

Disabled Sports USA of Northern California

The Unrecables (Los Angeles Chapter of Disabled Sports USA)

Adaptive Sports Center of Crested Butte (CO)

Breckenridge Outdoor Education Center (CO)

National Sports Center for the Disabled (CO)

Rocky Mountain Handicapped Sportsmen's Association (CO)

Baltimore Adapted Recreation and Sports (BARS) (MD)

Eagle Mount—Great Falls (MT)

I Am Third Foundation—dba Eagle Mount (MT)

Northeast Passage (NH)

Challenge New Mexico

Three Rivers Adaptive Sports (TRAS) (PA)

National Ability Center (UT)

Options for Independence (UT)

Richmond Athletes With Disabilities (RAD) Sports (VA)

ROCK CLIMBING

(*See* Climbing—Rock)

ROWING

Wheelchair Sports and Recreation (MA)

Disabled Sports USA—Lakeside Chapter (NV)

RUGBY

Sports Association, Gaylord Hospital (CT)

RIC Skiers—Wirtz Sports Program (IL)

Wheelchair Sports and Recreation (MA)

Disabled Sports USA—Lakeside Chapter (NV)

Disabled Sports Association of North Texas (TX)

Variety Wheelchair Arts and Sports Assn. (TX)

Richmond Athletes With Disabilities (RAD) Sports (VA)

RUGBY—QUAD

Sports Association, Gaylord Hospital (CT)

RIC Skiers—Wirtz Sports Program (IL)

Disabled Sports Association of North Texas (TX)

Richmond Athletes With Disabilities (RAD) Sports (VA)

SCUBA

Colorado Discover Ability

Sports Association, Gaylord Hospital (CT)

RIC Skiers—Wirtz Sports Program (IL)

Baltimore Adapted Recreation and Sports (BARS) (MD)

Wheelchair Sports and Recreation (MA)

Vermont Adaptive Ski and Sports Association

SAILING

Challenge Alaska Southeast

California Handicapped Skiers

Disabled Sports USA of Northern California

Sports Association, Gaylord Hospital (CT)

Judd Goldman Adaptive Sailing Program (IL)

Baltimore Adapted Recreation and Sports (BARS) (MD)

Chesapeake Region Accessible Boating (MD)

National Ocean Access Project (NOAP) (MD)

Community Boating (MA)

Courageous Sailing Center (MA)

Great Lakes Sailing Association for the Physically Disabled (MI)

New England Handicapped Sports (NH)

Sail-habilitation (NJ)

Sea Legs, The Disabled Sailing Experience (NY)

National Ocean Access Project, Houston Area Chapter (TX)

Variety Wheelchair Arts and Sports Assn. (TX)

Footloose Sailing Association (WA)

Operation Able/Sail (NB, Canada)

SELF-HELP

(*See* Personal Improvement)

SHOOTING—SKEET

Baltimore Adapted Recreation and Sports (BARS) (MD)

SHOOTING—TARGET

Northeast Passage (NH)

SKATING—ICE

Alpine Alternatives (AK)
Eagle Mount—Great Falls (MT)
Disabled Sports USA—Lakeside Chapter (NV)
Deutsch Institute (PA)
Variety Wheelchair Arts and Sports Assn. (TX)
Vermont Adaptive Ski and Sports Association

SKATING—ROLLER

Disabled Sports USA—Lakeside Chapter (NV)

SKIING—ALPINE

Alpine Alternatives (AK)
Challenge Alaska
Challenge Alaska, Kenai Peninsula
Challenge Alaska Southeast
Mesa Association of Sports for the Disabled (AZ)
California Handicapped Skiers
Disabled Sports USA of Northern California
The Unrecables (Los Angeles Chapter of Disabled Sports USA)
DS/USA Orange County Chapter ("The Achievers") (CA)
Mother Lode Chapter
Adaptive Sports Center of Crested Butte (CO)
Aspen Handicapped Skiers Association (CO)
Breckenridge Outdoor Education Center (CO)
Colorado Discover Ability
Adaptive Sports Association at Purgatory Resort (CO)
Eldora Special Recreation Program (ESRP) (CO)
National Sports Center for the Disabled (CO)
Southern Colorado Center for Challenged Athletes
Telluride Adaptive Ski Program (CO)
Connecticut Handicapped Ski Foundation
Sports Association, Gaylord Hospital (CT)
Nation's Capital Handicapped Sports (DC)
Disabled Sports USA—Atlanta Chapter (GA)

Recreation Unlimited (ID)

Chicagoland Handicapped Skiers (IL)

RIC Skiers—Wirtz Sports Program (IL)

Special Outdoor Leisure Opportunities (SOLO) (IN)

Maine Access-able Adventures

Maine Handicapped Skiing

Baltimore Adapted Recreation and Sports (BARS) (MD)

Cannonsburg Challenged Ski Association (MI)

Michigan Handicapped Sports & Recreation Association

Courage Center (MN)

Courage Duluth (MN)

Dream Disabled Ski Program (MT)

Eagle Mount—Great Falls (MT)

I Am Third Foundation—dba Eagle Mount (MT)

I Am Third Foundation—dba Eagle Mount—Billings (MT)

New England Handicapped Sports (NH)

Northeast Passage (NH)

Waterville Valley Foundation (NH)

The White Mountain Adaptive Ski School, Loon Mountain (NH)

The Adaptive Ski Program (NM)

Challenge New Mexico

Disabled Ski Program at Ski Windham (NY)

Greek Peak Sports for the Disabled (NY)

Lounsbury Adaptive Ski Program (NY)

Three Trackers of Ohio

Pennsylvania Center for Adapted Boats

Three Rivers Adaptive Sports (TRAS) (PA)

Amputees Coming Together of East Tennessee

National Ability Center (UT)

Options for Independence (UT)

Utah Handicapped Skiers Association

Vermont Adaptive Ski and Sports Association

Richmond Athletes With Disabilities (RAD) Sports (VA)

Disabled Sports USA Northwest ("Team USAble") (WA)

SKIING—NORDIC

Alpine Alternatives (AK)

Adaptive Sports Center of Crested Butte (CO)

Breckenridge Outdoor Education Center (CO)

Eldora Special Recreation Program (ESRP) (CO)

National Sports Center for the Disabled (CO)
RIC Skiers—Wirtz Sports Program (IL)
Maine Handicapped Skiing
I Am Third Foundation—dba Eagle Mount (MT)
Northeast Passage (NH)
Waterville Valley Foundation (NH)
Amputees Coming Together of East Tennessee

SKIING—WATER

Challenge Alaska
California Handicapped Skiers
Disabled Sports USA of Northern California
The Unrecables (Los Angeles Chapter of Disabled Sports USA)
Nation's Capital Handicapped Sports (DC)
Physically Adapted Recreation and Sports (FL)
Baltimore Adapted Recreation and Sports (BARS) (MD)
Michigan Handicapped Sports & Recreation Association
Courage Center (MN)
Disabled Sports USA—Lakeside Chapter (NV)
Northeast Passage (NH)
Three Trackers of Ohio
Three Rivers Adaptive Sports (TRAS) (PA)
Variety Wheelchair Arts and Sports Assn. (TX)
National Ability Center (UT)
Vermont Adaptive Ski and Sports Association
Richmond Athletes With Disabilities (RAD) Sports (VA)

SLEDDING—DOG

Challenge Alaska
Options for Independence (UT)
Vermont Adaptive Ski and Sports Association

SLEDDING—ICE

Wheelchair Sports and Recreation (MA)
Northeast Passage (NH)
Vermont Adaptive Ski and Sports Association

SLEDGING—ICE

Vermont Adaptive Ski and Sports Association

SNOWMOBILING

Challenge Alaska
Disabled Sports USA—Lakeside Chapter (NV)

SNOWSHOEING

Breckenridge Outdoor Education Center (CO)
(*See also* Winter Sports)

SOFTBALL—GENERAL

Disabled Sports USA—Lakeside Chapter (NV)

SOFTBALL—WHEELCHAIR

RIC Skiers—Wirtz Sports Program (IL)

SPORTS—COMPETITIVE

Challenge Alaska

National Sports Center for the Disabled (CO)

Northeast Passage (NH)

A.S.P.I.R.E. (New York/Long Island)

Sea Legs, The Disabled Sailing Experience (NY)

STRENGTH AND CONDITIONING

RIC Skiers—Wirtz Sports Program (IL)

Northeast Passage (NH)

Warriors on Wheels (NY)

Disabled Sports Association of North Texas (TX)

SUMMER SPORTS

Sports, Arts, and Recreation of Chattanooga (TN)

SWIMMING

Mesa Association of Sports for the Disabled (AZ)

RIC Skiers—Wirtz Sports Program (IL)

Wheelchair Sports and Recreation (MA)

Eagle Mount—Great Falls (MT)

I Am Third Foundation—dba Eagle Mount-Billings (MT)

Disabled Sports USA—Lakeside Chapter (NV)

Disabled Sports Association of North Texas (TX)

Variety Wheelchair Arts and Sports Assn. (TX)

National Ability Center (UT)

Vermont Adaptive Ski and Sports Association

Richmond Athletes With Disabilities (RAD) Sports (VA)

TENNIS—GENERAL

Sports Association, Gaylord Hospital (CT)

RIC Skiers—Wirtz Sports Program (IL)

Wheelchair Sports and Recreation (MA)

Disabled Sports USA—Lakeside Chapter (NV)

Waterville Valley Foundation (NH)

Challenge New Mexico

Deutsch Institute (PA)

Three Rivers Adaptive Sports (TRAS) (PA)

Variety Wheelchair Arts and Sports Assn. (TX)

National Ability Center (UT)

TENNIS—TABLE

Disabled Sports USA—Lakeside Chapter (NV)

Variety Wheelchair Arts and Sports Assn. (TX)

TRACK AND FIELD

Physically Adapted Recreation and Sports (FL)

Wheelchair Sports and Recreation (MA)

Disabled Sports USA—Lakeside Chapter (NV)

A.S.P.I.R.E. (New York/Long Island)

Disabled Sports Association of North Texas (TX)

Variety Wheelchair Arts and Sports Assn. (TX)

TENNIS—WHEELCHAIR

Baltimore Adapted Recreation and Sports (BARS) (MD)

A.S.P.I.R.E. (Upstate New York)

Disabled Sports Association of North Texas (TX)

Richmond Athletes With Disabilities (RAD) Sports (VA)

VOLLEYBALL—GENERAL

Disabled Sports USA—Lakeside Chapter (NV)

Deutsch Institute (PA)

Variety Wheelchair Arts and Sports Assn. (TX)

VOLLEYBALL—SITTING

RIC Skiers—Wirtz Sports Program (IL)

WATER WEIGHTS

(*See* Powerlifting and Weightlifting)

WEIGHTLIFTING

(*See* Powerlifting and Weightlifting)

WEIGHT TRAINING

(*See* Powerlifting and Weightlifting)

WHEELCHAIR SPORTS

Breckenridge Outdoor Education Center (CO)

Wheelchair Sports and Recreation (MA)

Northeast Passage (NH)

Warriors on Wheels (NY)

Variety Wheelchair Arts and Sports Assn. (TX)

Richmond Athletes With Disabilities (RAD) Sports (VA)
    (*See also* Basketball—Wheelchair, Billiards—Wheelchair, Hockey—
    Wheelchair, Softball—Wheelchair, Tennis—Wheelchair)

Wilderness Experiences

Alpine Alternatives (AK)

Breckenridge Outdoor Education Center (CO)

Disabled Sports USA—Lakeside Chapter (NV)

Paraplegics on Independent Nature Trips (POINT) (TX)

National Ability Center (UT)

Windsurfing

United States Integrated Windsurfing (MA)

Winter Sports

RIC Skiers—Wirtz Sports Program (IL)

Northeast Passage (NH)

Sports, Arts, and Recreation of Chattanooga (TN)
    (*See also* Skiing—Alpine, Skiing—Nordic, Sledding, Snowshoeing)

Wrestling

Wheelchair Sports and Recreation (MA)

Disabled Sports USA—Lakeside Chapter (NV)

Yoga

Northeast Passage (NH)

Richmond Athletes With Disabilities (RAD) Sports (VA)

Youth Programs and Sports

Warriors on Wheels (NY)

Disabled Sports Association of North Texas (TX)

Organizations by State

Alabama

Alabama Handicapped Sportsmen
11802 Creighton Avenue
Northport, AL 35476
    Phone: (205)339-2800
    Contact: David Sullivan
    Program: Hunting

ALASKA

Alpine Alternatives, Inc.
2518 East Tudor Road, Suite 105
Anchorage, AK 99507

Phones: (907)561-6655; (907)563-9232 Fax

Contact: Margaret Webber

Programs: Summer camps varying in duration from three to seven days, equestrian programs, alpine and nordic skiing, canoeing, hiking, ice skating, wilderness experiences

Recreational Equipment: Sit-skis, ski bridges, outriggers, canoes

Challenge Alaska
P.O. Box 110065
Anchorage, AK 99511-0065

Phones: (907)563-2658; (907)561-6142 Fax

Contact: Mark Whitehurst

Programs: Winter program includes recreational and competitive alpine skiing at Alyeska Resort, dog sledding, snowmobiling, cabin camping, fitness classes and various social and leisure activities such as ice hockey games, museums, parties and cultural events. Summer programs include fishing, river rafting, water-skiing, canoeing, rock climbing, camping, deep sea fishing, and sea kayaking. Custom designed adventures are also available.

Major Events: Ski-A-Thon, Glacier Dash, Million Dollar Golf Shootout, Homer Halibut Fishing

Publication: Challenge Alaska, semi-annually.

Recreational Equipment: All downhill ski equipment, kayaks, and canoes. Fishing, water-skiing, rock climbing, and camping equipment

Challenge Alaska, Kenai Peninsula
P.O. Box 3638
Soldotna, AK 99699

Phones: (907)260-3804; (907)260-2676 Fax

Contact: Leslie Roberts

Programs: Downhill skiing, fishing, camping, and social events.

Major Event: Ski-A-Thon

Recreational Equipment: Fishing gear, tents

Challenge Alaska Southeast
P.O. Box 35134
Juneau, AK 99803-5134

Phones: (907)789-9747; (907)561-6142 Fax

Contact: Maureen Riley

Programs: Skiing, kayaking, sailing, biking, and camping

Recreational Equipment: Downhill skiing equipment, kayaks, canoes, fishing and camping equipment.

ARIZONA

Mesa Association of Sports for the Disabled
P.O. Box 4727
Mesa, AZ 85211-4727

Phones: (602)649-2194; (602)649-2258 Fax

Contact: Gregg Baumgarten

Programs: 18 Special Olympic sports; 8 sports for physically challenged; disabled skiing program

Major Events:

Event	Month
Desert Challenge Games	March
Mesa Swim Challenge	October
Learn to Ski/SkiAbilities	December
Mesa Bowling Challenge	December

Publication: Sportsline, Circulation 700, 4x/year

Recreational Equipment: Mono-ski, bi-ski, ski bra, bocce and bowling ramps, racing chairs.

CALIFORNIA

California Handicapped Skiers
P.O. Box 2897
Big Bear Lake, CA 92315

Phones: (909)585-2519, ext. 269; (909)585-6805 Fax

Contact: Kelle Malkewitz

Programs: California Adapted Ski School (alpine ski lessons), Alpine Challenge (camping and instruction for water-skiing, kayaking, canoeing, fishing, sailing, and personal water craft use).

Major Events:

Event	Month
Don Diego Ski Club Silent Auction	November
Ski-A-Thon	February
PSIA Instructor Certification	Annual
Sunday Scramble Golf Tournament	July

Publication: CHS Spirit, Circulation 6000, 4x/year

Recreational Equipment: Mono-and bi-skis, ski bras, Kawasaki Jet Skis, kayaks, pontoon boats, camping equipment

Disabled Sports USA of Northern California
6060 Sunrise Vista Drive, Suite 3030
Citrus Heights, CA 95610

Phones: (916)722-6447; (916)722-2627 Fax

Contact: Brian Quinn

Web Site: http://members.aol.com/jheycke/tass.htm

Programs: Winter Program: Tahoe Adaptive Ski School;

Summer Program: Operation Challenge—regional water-ski camps, kayaking, canoeing, sailing, camping, whitewater rafting, traveling water-ski clinics

Publication: Ventures, Circulation 3000, 2x/year

Recreational Equipment: Adapted snow-skiing and water-skiing equipment.

DS/USA Orange County Chapter
22361 Pine Glen
Mission Viejo, CA 92692

Phones: (714)586-7754; (714)581-5809 Fax

Contacts: Rob and Sharon Mitchell

Program: Snow-skiing instruction

Major Event: Ski-A-Thon in April

Publication: The Achievements, monthly newsletter

Recreational Equipment: Bi-, mono-, and sit-skis

Mother Lode Chapter
P.O. Box 4274
Camp Connell, CA 95223

Phones: (209)795-5811; (209)795-4423 Fax

Contact: Rick Van Aken

Program: Adapted alpine ski program

Major Events: Gala dinner/dance; David Brauer Race; Bear Valley Wine, Art and Beer Dance

Publication: Newsletter

Recreational Equipment: Adaptive ski equipment

The Unrecables (Los Angeles Chapter of Disabled Sports USA)
(Formerly DS/USA of Southern California)
P.O. Box 24856
Los Angeles, CA 90024-0856

E-mail: unrecables@earthlink.net

Phones: (310)823-1373; (310)838-6213 Fax

Contact: Sigrid Noack, President (1996-97) - (310)823-1373
Gordon W. Cardona, Vice President (1996-97) - (213)283-4414

Web Site: http://home.earthlink.net/~unrecables/

Programs: Downhill skiing at Mammoth Mountain, whitewater rafting, camping, water-skiing, Hollywood Bowl, concerts, and parties

Social Meetings: Every second Tuesday of each month at 7: 00 P.M. at the V.A. Medical Center, Building 500, 11301 Wilshire Bl., L.A.

Publication: Newsletter

Recreational Equipment: Mono-skis, bi-skis, sit-skis, kayaks, water skis and life jackets

COLORADO

Adaptive Sports Center of Crested Butte
P.O. Box 1639
Crested Butte, CO 81224

Phones: (970)349-2296; (970)349-2250 Fax

Contacts: Chris Hensley or Mary Manion

Programs: Alpine and nordic skiing, rock climbing, horseback riding, "back-country trips," whitewater rafting, and mountain biking

Major Events: "Free Ski"—lift tickets for members are free for four weeks (late November-mid-December), winter sports clinics for Disabled American Veterans (DAV)

Publication: Quarterly newsletter

Recreational Equipment: Adaptive skiing equipment

Aspen Handicapped Skiers Association
Box E-2
Snowmass Village, CO 81615

Phone: (970)923-4269

Contact: Charles Racine

Program: Alpine skiing

Breckenridge Outdoor Education Center
P.O. Box 697
Breckenridge, CO 80424

Phones: (970)453-6422; (970)453-4676 Fax

Contact: Lisa Reed

Programs: Alpine and Nordic skiing, snowshoeing, climbing, canoeing, camping, backpacking, wilderness courses, rafting, extended river trips, mountaineering, extended river trips, teambuilding and "Professional Challenge" programs. Ski-in lodging for groups.

Major Event: Host chapter for DS/USA'S SKI SPECTACULAR

Publication: Empowering News, Circulation 5000, 2x/year

Recreational Equipment: Adaptive ski equipment, wheelchair-accessible ropes course and climbing wall

Colorado Discover Ability
P.O. Box 3444
Grand Junction, CO 81501

Phones: (970)268-5700; (970)874-3002 Fax

Contact: Linda Vickers

Programs: Ski program at Powderhorn, scuba diving

Major Events: Ski race, golf tournament

Recreational Equipment: Bi-skis, mono-skis, outriggers

Adaptive Sports Association at Purgatory Resort
P.O. Box 1884
Durango, CO 81302

Phones: (970)259-0374; (970)259-2175 Fax

Contact: Eleanor Guerrero

Program: Adaptive ski school

Major Events:

Event	Month
Ski Swap	October
Ski-A-Thon	January
Pro Football Players' Race	February
Beer Fest	September

Recreational Equipment: Adaptive ski equipment, including mono-skis, bi-skis, and outriggers

Eldora Special Recreation Program (ESRP)

P.O. Box 19106

Boulder, CO 80308

Phones: (303)442-0606; (303)440-5752 Fax

Contact: Jane Owen

Programs: Nordic and alpine skiing

Major Event: Special Olympics ski race

Recreational Equipment: Adaptive ski equipment for nordic and alpine skiing, ski racing equipment

Golf 4 Fun

P.O. Box 5304

Englewood, CO 80155

Phones: (303)985-3403; (303)988-8133

Contact: Bob Nelson

Program: Golf lessons from PGA professionals

Major Events: Annual Golf 4 Fun tournament, Annual Play Day for students and volunteers

Publication: The Links Letter, Circulation 600, 2x/year

Recreational Equipment: Golf clubs

National Sports Center for the Disabled

P.O. Box 36

Winter Park, CO 80482

Phones: (970)726-1548; (970)726-4112 Fax

Contact: Paul DiBello

Web Site: http://www.nscd.org/nscd/

Programs: Competitive alpine ski racing, rock climbing, nordic skiing, white water rafting, mountain biking, hiking and camping, fishing, and miniature golf

Major Events:

Event	Month
First Interstate Bank Cup	February
Annual Spring Dinner	March
Hal O'Leary Golf Classic	July
Wine, Beer, Food Festival	August

Publications: Bold Tracks, worldwide sales, Every three years; Outrigger, Circulation 10,000, 4x/year

Recreational Equipment: Alpine and nordic adaptive ski equipment, hand-cranked bikes, mountain bikes (single and tandem), camping and fishing equipment

Rocky Mountain Handicapped Sportsmen's Association
Box 18036 Capitol Hill Station
Denver, CO 80218
Phone: (303)934-9540
Contact: Tom Reetz
Program: Whitewater rafting

Southern Colorado Center for Challenged Athletes
25069 Road BB
La Junta, CO 81050
Phone: (719)384-6580
Contact: Royce A. Miller, P.T.
Program: Alpine skiing

Telluride Adaptive Ski Program
P.O. Box 2254
Telluride, CO 81435
Phone: (970)728-7537
Contact: Norm Benjamin
Program: Adaptive alpine skiing

CONNECTICUT

Connecticut Handicapped Ski Foundation
52 Whaleas Point
East Haven, CT 06512
Phone: (203)468-2145
Contact: Karen Smith
Program: Alpine skiing

Sports Association, Gaylord Hospital
Therapeutic Recreation Department
Box 400
Wallingford, CT 06492
Phone: (203)284-2800, x 3424
Contact: Ken Murphy
Programs: Ski club, archery, tennis and golf clinics, wheelchair basketball, Connecticut Jammers quad rugby club, aerobics, "soaring discovery nights," scuba diving, sailing, golf club
Major Events: Gaylord Fitness Festival, Five-Mile Road Race, Northeast Regional Quad Rugby Tournament
Recreational Equipment: Adaptive downhill ski equipment, golfing equipment, archery equipment, rackets, golf driving range, and adapted golf cart

DISTRICT OF COLUMBIA

Nation's Capital Handicapped Sports
P.O. Box 76760
Washington, DC 20013
Phone: (301)498-5564
Contact: June Friedman
Programs: Water-skiing, adaptive skiing at Whitetail, PA
Major Events: Halloween 5K and 10K run (conducted with DS/USA's national office)

FLORIDA

c/o Memorial Regional Rehabilitation Center
P.O. Box 16406
Jacksonville, FL 32245-6406
Phones: (904)858-7277; (904)858-7619 Fax
Contact: Janet Collins
Programs: water-skiing, track and field, social events

GEORGIA

Disabled Sports USA—Atlanta Chapter
P.O. Box 327
Clarkston, GA 30021
Phone: (404)498-7204
Contact: Stacy McPherson
Program: Alpine skiing

IDAHO

Recreation Unlimited
3131 Chinden Blvd
Boise, ID 83714
Phones: (208)345-1822; (208)362-5869 Fax
Contact: Virginia Collier
Program: Alpine ski instruction
Recreational Equipment: Mono-skis, bi-skis, sit-skis, outriggers

ILLINOIS

Chicagoland Handicapped Skiers
1086 Briarcliffe
Wheaton, IL 60187
Phone: (708)682-4018
Contact: Bud Sanders
Program: Alpine skiing

Judd Goldman Adaptive Sailing Program
Chicago Park District
425 East McFetridge Drive
Chicago, IL 60605

Phones: (312)747-0737; (312)747-7684; (312)747-6598 Fax

Contact: Ted Sutherland

Programs: Sailing lessons which include race training, custom sailing programs, and boat rentals

Major Events: North American Challenge Cup and Independence Cup (National Championships for disabled sailing, conducted with U.S. Sailing); Goldman Cup; Freedom Cup; Foundation benefit dinner

Recreational Equipment: Freedom Independence (specially adapted sailboat for paraplegics and quadriplegics), other sailboats

RIC Skiers—Wirtz Sports Program
Rehabilitation Institute of Chicago
345 E. Superior Street
Chicago, IL 60611

Phones: (312)908-4292; (312)908-1051 Fax

Contact: Jeff Jones

Programs: Aerobics, basketball, quad rugby, powerlifting, sitting volleyball, strength and conditioning, swimming, tennis, fencing, golf, scuba diving, wheelchair softball, and winter sports

Major Events:

Event	Month
Wheelchair Basketball Tournament	December
Annual Road Race	September
Annual Hole-in-One	June

Publication: RIC Sports Report, monthly

INDIANA

Special Outdoor Leisure Opportunities (SOLO), Inc.
P.O. Box 6221
South Bend, IN 46660

Phones: (219)237-5252; (219)237-5520 Fax

Contacts: Ellen and Dave Grinnel

Program: Alpine Skiing

MAINE

Maine Access-able Adventures
P.O. Box 3817
Portland, ME 04104

Phone: (207)871-2993

Contact: Joellen Ross

Programs: Horseback riding, bicycle riding, kayaking, canoeing, and rock climbing.

Major Event: Ski Weekend

Publication: Seasonal calendar of events

Maine Handicapped Skiing
RR 2, Box 1971, Sunday River Ski Resort
Bethel, ME 04217

Phones: (800)639-7770; (207)824-2440; (207)824-2440 Fax

Contact: Paula Wheeler

Programs: Adaptive alpine and nordic skiing

Major Event: Ski-A-Thon

Recreational Equipment: Mono-skis, bi-skis, sit-skis, outriggers, walkers

MARYLAND

Baltimore Adapted Recreation and Sports (BARS)
P.O. Box 878
Sparks, MD 21152

Phones: (410)472-3363; (410)472-3363 Fax

Contact: Pamela Harris-Lehnert

Programs: Water-skiing, snow-skiing, canoeing, sailing, scuba diving, skeet shooting, wheelchair tennis, racquetball, hand cycling, kayaking, nature walks, rafting, and camping

Publication: Quarterly newsletter

Recreational Equipment: Bi-skis, mono-skis, water skis, kayaks, sailboats, tents

Chesapeake Region Accessible Boating
P.O. Box 6564
Annapolis, MD 21401-0564

Phone: (410)974-2628

Contact: Don Backe

Programs: Adapted sailing, "Sail Free" clinics the last Sunday of each month, May-September. Private lessons available. Call for details.

National Ocean Access Project (NOAP)
P.O. Box 1705
Rockville, MD 20849-1705

Phones: (301)217-9843; (301)217-9843 Fax

Contact: Stephen Spinetto

Programs: Regional sailing programs at NOAP chapters nationwide and in Canada

Major Events: Assist U.S. Sailing in conduct of Independence Cup (national disabled yachting regatta). Conducted 1993 World Disabled Sailing Championships with Disabled Sports USA.

Recreational Equipment: Maintain information on adapted sailing equipment such as the Freedom Independence Sailboat, and adapted sailing seat for paraplegic and quadriplegic sailors

MASSACHUSETTS

Community Boating
21 Embankment Road
Boston, MA 02114
> *Phone:* (617)523-1038
> *Contact:* Bill Pendleton
> *Program:* Adaptive sailing

Courageous Sailing Center
1 First Avenue
Charlestown Navy Yard, Parris Building
Charlestown, MA 02129
> *Phone:* (617)725-3263
> *Contact:* Dru Slattery
> *Program:* Adaptive sailing

United States Integrated Windsurfing
119 High Street
Acton, MA 01720
> *Phone:* (508)263-2332
> *Contact:* Ross Lilley
> *Programs:* Windsurfing lessons are offered in Boston and Rhode Island.
> *Recreational Equipment:* Windsurfing catamarans, seats, harnesses, hearing devices

Wheelchair Sports and Recreation Association, Inc.
2001 Marina Drive, #113
North Quincy, MA 02171
> *Phone:* (617)773-7251
> *Contact:* Charles Ekizian
> *Programs:* Powerlifting, rugby, scuba diving, swimming, wrestling, fitness, basketball, cycling, fishing, ice sledding, racquetball, rowing, tennis, weightlifting, canoeing, hunting, kayaking, martial arts, pentathlon, sledge hockey, track and field, handcycling (*See also* The White Mountain Adaptive Ski School, Loon Mountain (NH) based in Boston, MA.)

MICHIGAN

Cannonsburg Challenged Ski Association
P.O. Box 14, 6800 Cannonsburg Road
Cannonsburg, MI 49317
> *Phones:* (616)453-0320; (616)453-0750 Fax
> *Contact:* Jean Weygandt
> *Programs:* Downhill skiing and canoeing
> *Major Events:*

Event	Month
Take the Challenge ski race	February
PSIA-adapted instructor certification	January

Publication: Newsletter

Recreational Equipment: Mono-skis, bi-skis, outriggers, adaptive canoe seats

Great Lakes Sailing Association for the Physically Disabled
150 West Jefferson, Suite 900
Detroit, MI 48220
  Phone: (313)822-3019
  Contact: Dan Rustman
  Program: Adapted sailing

Michigan Handicapped Sports & Recreation Association
P.O. Box 240368
Orchard Lake, MI 48324-0368
  Phones: (810)682-3966; (810)362-1702 Fax
  Contacts: Carol Roubal or Chet Kuskowski
  Programs: Snow-skiing and racing, water-skiing
  Publication: Newsletter
  Recreational Equipment: Mono-skis, bi-skis, 3- and 4-track ski equipment

MINNESOTA

Courage Center
3915 Golden Valley Road
Golden Valley, MN 55422
  Phones: (612)520-0479; (612)520-0577 Fax
  Contact: Tobe Broadrick
  Programs: Snow-skiing and water-skiing
  Publication: Yearly calendar
  Recreational Equipment: Archery equipment, snow skis, water skis

Courage Duluth
205 West 2nd Street #200
Duluth, MN 55804
  Phones: (218)727-0430; (218)727-2874 Fax
  Contact: Eric Larson
  Program: Downhill skiing
  Publication: Seasonal program brochure
  Recreational Equipment: Basketball wheelchairs, ski and archery equipment

U.S. Electric Wheelchair Hockey Association
7216 39th Avenue North
New Hope, MN 55427
  Phone: (612)535-4736
  Contact: Craig McClellan
  Program: Wheelchair hockey

MONTANA

Dream Disabled Ski Program
P.O. Box 8300
Kalispell, MT 59904-8300

Phones: (406)758-5411; (406)756-6582 Fax

Contact: Sandra Center

Program: Alpine skiing program which offers one-on-one skiing instruction

Major Events:

Events	Month
Montana Special Olympics	March
Ski Pledge Mania fundraiser	February

Recreational Equipment: Bi-skis, mono-skis, 3- and 4-track ski equipment, sit-skis

Eagle Mount—Great Falls
4237 Second Avenue North
Great Falls, MT 59401

Phones: (406)454-1449; (406)454-1780 Fax

Contact: Tina Hlad

Programs: Hiking, horseback riding, ice skating, swimming, aquatic aerobics, rafting, children's day camp, alpine skiing

I Am Third Foundation—dba Eagle Mount
6901 Goldenstein Ln.
Bozeman, MT 59715

Phones: (406)586-1781; (406)586-5794 Fax

Contact: Linda Griffith

Programs: Nordic and downhill skiing, aquatic therapy and aquatic golf, horseback riding, horticulture, rafting and day trips

Major Event: Ride-A-Thon in August

I Am Third Foundation—dba Eagle Mount—Billings
2822 3rd Avenue North, Suite 203
Billings, MT 59101

Phones: (406)245-5422; (406)245-5529 Fax

Contact: Deborah Speer

Programs: Summer activities, snow-skiing, golfing, hunting, and swimming

Major Events:

Event	Month
Swim-A-Thon	October
Warren Miller movie	November
EagleFest	March

Recreational Equipment: Adaptive skiing, golfing, and swimming equipment

NEVADA

Disabled Sports USA—Lakeside Chapter
749 Veterans Memorial Drive
Las Vegas, NV 89101

Phone: (702)229-6297

Contact: Roy Rost

Programs: Wrestling, track and field, water polo, mountain climbing, road racing, softball, table tennis, all-terrain vehicles, canoeing, gardening, gymnastics, hiking, ice skating, martial arts, baseball, handball, horseback riding, judo, lawn bowls, powerlifting, roller skating, rugby, snowmobiling, swimming, tae kwan do, trampoline and tumbling, water-skiing, fitness, wilderness experiences, basketball, cycling, fishing, football, gold, karate, racquetball, rowing, tennis, volleyball, weightlifting, bowling.

New Hampshire

New England Handicapped Sports Association (NEHSA)
P.O. Box 2135
Mt. Sunapee, NH 03255-2135

Phone: (800)628-4484 Voice/Fax

Contact: Amy Lane

Programs: Snow-skiing, canoe trip, and golf

Major Events:

Event	Month
Ski-a-Thon	February
Corporate challenge race	March
Regional skiing race	January
Golf tournament	September

Publications: Quarterly newsletter, yearly brochure

Recreational Equipment: Adaptive skiing equipment and sailboats

Northeast Passage
P.O. Box 127
Durham, NH 03824

Phones: (603)862-0070; (603)862-2722 Fax

Contact: Jill Gravink

Programs: 10 instructional clinics in different sports each year (e.g. sea kayaking, water-skiing, conditioning, racquetball, target shooting); 4 accessible vacations that vary based on participant interest (e.g., whitewater rafting, wellness, yoga, massage, tai chi); sports development (including organized/competitive sled hockey, wheelchair sports camp for kids); resource referral through computerized database

Recreational Equipment: Mono-skis, bi-skis, cross-country sit-skis, ice sleds, handcycles, water skis, knobby tired wheelchairs, racing chairs, beach access fence

Waterville Valley Foundation
Adaptive Sports Programs
Box 464
Waterville Valley, NH 03215

Phones: (603)236-8311, x 5500; (603)236-4344 Fax

Contact: Kathy Chandler

Programs: Alpine skiing, tennis, golf, nordic skiing

Major Events: Since 1993, Eastern Regional Disabled Ski Championships (final eastern race in regional qualifying series for U.S. Disabled Ski Championships)

Recreational Equipment: Adaptive downhill ski equipment

The White Mountain Adaptive Ski School, Loon Mountain (NH)
55 Washington Avenue
Boston MA 02152

Phones: (603)745-8111, x 5663; (603)745-8214 Fax

Contact: Robert Harney, M.D.

Programs: Adaptive ski instruction and race clinics offered; summer programs are currently in developmental stages

Major Event: Kostick Kup race

Publication: DS/USA Update

Recreational Equipment: Adaptive ski equipment

NEW JERSEY

Sail-habilitation
9 Hospital Drive
Toms River, NJ 08755

Phone: (908)505-5115; (908)505-1817 Fax

Contact: Dr. Stephanie P. Argyris

NEW MEXICO

The Adaptive Ski Program
2425 Ridgecrest Drive, S.E.
Albuquerque, NM 87108

Phones: (800)877-7526; (505)262-7563; (505)262-7598 Fax

Contact: Karen White

Programs: Skiing and ski racing

Major Events:

Event	Month
Celebrity Ski Challenge	February
Beer-tasting Fundraiser	May

Publication: The Ski Link, Circulation 500, 4x/year

Recreational Equipment: Mono-skis, bi-skis, sit-skis, and 3/4 track

Challenge New Mexico
1570 Pacheco #E-6
Santa Fe, NM 87501

Phones: (505)988-7621; (505)988-9164 Fax

Contact: Chris Werhane

Programs: Horseback riding, skiing, tennis, rafting, Little League, and basketball

Major Event: Ride-a-Thon in October

Recreational Equipment: Horseback, skiing, tennis, rafting, basketball, and base-ball equipment

New York

A.S.P. I.R.E. (New York/Long Island)
50 Maple Place
Manhasset, NY 11031

Phones: (516)627-3996; (516)365-7225; (516)365-7112 Fax

Contact: Paddy Rossbach

Programs: Self-help support groups, track training. sport-specific training, and junior competition training

A.S.P. I.R.E. (Upstate New York)
P.O. Box 2042
Albany, NY 12220

Phones: (518)374-6011; (518)393-3292 Fax

Contact: Thomas Swank

Programs: Amputees and spinal cord injured on call

Major Events:

Event	Month
World Wheelchair Tennis Tournament	July
Wheelchair Tennis Clinic	July
Fitness Clinic	Spring

Publications: Nonprofit Organization directory, newsletter

Disabled Ski Program at Ski Windham
c/o EPSIA Educational Foundation
1-A Lincoln Avenue
Albany, NY 12205

Phones: (518)452-6095; (518)452-6099 Fax

Contact: Gwen Allard

Programs: Race program and instructor training

Major Events:

Event	Month
Dinner Dance/Silent Auction	February
Disabled Festival Weekend	March
Golf Tournament	May-August

Publication: Biannual newsletter

Recreational Equipment: Bi-skis, mono-skis, and outriggers

Greek Peak Sports for the Disabled
508 Verna Drive
Endwell, NY 13760

Phones: (607)785-6960; (607)729-6271

Contact: Dick Wierman

Program: Alpine skiing

Publication: Annual newsletter

Lounsbury Adaptive Ski Program
Holiday Valley, P.O. Box 370
Ellicottville, NY 14731

Phones: (716)699-2345; (716)871-8295; (716)699-5204 Fax

Contact: Jane Probst

Web Site: http://www.nornet.on.ca/~bfitz/ski.html

Program: Ski lessons, by appointment, are offered daily

Major Events: Penguin Paddle fundraiser, BBQ, races

Publication: A volunteer manual is published yearly

Recreational Equipment: Mono-skis, bi-skis, sit-skis, outriggers

Sea Legs, The Disabled Sailing Experience
P.O. Box 2011
New York, NY 10159-2011

E-mail: hfletch@aol.com

Phones: (212)645-7245; (212)263-8566 Fax

Contact: Honey Shields

Web Site: http://www.gorp.com/nonprof/sealegs/

Programs: Recreational and competitive sailing, and sailing lessons

Major Events:

Event	Month
Sail-a-Thon	September
Sailabration	June

Publication: The Captain's Log, Circulation 600, 2x/year

Recreational Equipment: Adaptive sailing equipment

Warriors on Wheels
409 Hackett Boulevard
Albany, NY 12208

Phone: (518)453-9205

Contact: Ned Norton

Programs: Strength training for individuals with disabilities, emphasis on weight training, junior program for youth

Publication: Exercise video: "Strength Training for Independence"

OHIO

Three Trackers of Ohio
2024 Rossmoor Road
Cleveland Heights, OH 44118-2515

Phones: (216)243-4068 or (216)371-1674; (216)778-5206 Fax, attn: Jackie Otte

Contact: Yolanda Niemoller

Programs: Downhill ski instruction and racing, biking, and golfing

Major Events: Three Trackers of Ohio's Ski Spectacular; Operation Challenge (water-skiing)

Publication: Monthly newsletter

Recreational Equipment: Major inventory of adaptive downhill ski equipment

PENNSYLVANIA

Deutsch Institute
615 Jefferson Avenue, Suite 201
Scranton, PA 18510

Phones: (717)348-1968; (717)348-4774 Fax

Contact: Dave Klein

Programs: Ice skating, tennis clinics, therapeutic recreation and leisure workshops, bowling leagues

Major Events:

Event	Month
Wheelchair billiards tournament	March
Summer day camp for children	July-Aug

Publication: Pocono NE Digest, Circulation 1700, 4x/year

Recreational Equipment: Bowling ramps, basketballs, tennis racquets, volleyballs, bocce, and many, many games

Pennsylvania Center for Adapted Boats
#4 Boathouse Row, Kelly Drive
Philadelphia, PA 19130

Phones: (215)765-5118; (215)765-4504 Fax

Contact: Isabel Bohn

Program: Adaptive snow-skiing at Jack Frost Mountain, Poconos, PA

Recreational Equipment: Mono-skis, bi-skis, (adult and children), outriggers

Three Rivers Adaptive Sports (TRAS)
P.O. Box 38235
Pittsburgh, PA 15238

Phones: (412)749-2281 or (412)561-1569; (412)749-2323 Fax

Contact: Mark Kulzer

Programs: Adaptive snow ski instruction, water ski instruction, camping trips, canoeing, rafting, paintball, hay rides, tennis, cycling, sea-kayaking, wheelchair basketball, social events, and bowling

Major Events: Bowl-A-Thon, Learn to Ski clinics (water and snow)

Publication: Monthly newsletter

Recreational Equipment: Adaptive snow ski equipment, Kan Skis, cages, outriggers, quick releases, Deep V Ropes, hand cycles, canoes, rafts, camping equipment

TENNESSEE

Amputees Coming Together of East Tennessee
c/o Orthopedic Associates
1932 Alcoa Highway
Knoxville, TN 37920

Phone: (423)524-8772

Contact: Mike Rollo

Programs: Adaptive alpine and nordic skiing

Major Event: Ski-A-Thon

Recreational Equipment: Mono-skis, bi-skis, sit-skis, outriggers, walkers

Program: Children's amputee camp

Publication: Monthly newsletter

Sports, Arts and Recreation of Chattanooga
4713 Bonny Oaks Drive, #2403
Chattanooga, TN 37416

Phone: (615)899-6255

Contact: Cathy Fletcher

Programs: A variety of summer and winter sports, and theater trips

TEXAS

Amputee Connection Inc., dba Just a Little Inconvenience
P.O. Box 4
Portland, TX 78374

Phone: (512)643-8904 Voice/Fax

Program: Basketball

Disabled Sports Association of North Texas, Inc.
3810 West Northwest Highway, Suite 205
Dallas, TX 75330

Phones: (214)352-4100; (214)352-1744 Fax

Contact: Kim Kavanagh

Programs: Track and field, bocce, swimming, soccer, bowling, strength and conditioning, wheelchair basketball, wheelchair tennis, team handball, quad rugby, and youth sports clubs

Major Events: Western National Wheelchair Tennis Champs; Youth Challenge (developmental track meet)

Publication: Sports Page, Circulation 1,500, 4x/year

National Ocean Access Project, Houston Area Chapter
11603 Orchard Mountain Drive
Houston, TX 77059

Phone: (713)334-1993

Contact: Larry Smith

Program: Sailing

Paraplegics on Independent Nature Trips (POINT)
4144 North Central Expressway, Suite 515
Dallas, TX 75204

Phones: (214)827-7404; (214)851-7476 Fax

Contact: Jules Brenner

Major Event: National Handicapped Bass Tournament

Variety Wheelchair Arts and Sports Assn.
4144 N. Central Expwy., #130
Dallas, TX 75204

Phone: (214)495-6508

Contact: Carol Barrett

Programs: Horseback riding, rugby, swimming, water-skiing, fitness, archery, basketball, bicycling, camping, fishing, football, soccer, tennis, triathlon, volleyball, weightlifting, bowling, canoeing, fencing, ice skating, kayaking, martial arts, road racing, sailing, table tennis, track and field

Utah

National Ability Center
P.O. Box 682799
Park City, UT 84068

Phones: (801)649-3991; (801)649-3991 Fax

Contact: Meeche White

Web Site: http://www.utahrec.com/NAC.htm

Programs: Horseback riding, outdoor education, rafting, water-skiing, swimming, snow-skiing, basketball, hiking, wilderness experiences, camping, fishing, golf, and tennis

Major Event: Huntsman's Cup in January

Publication: Ability Bulletin, Circulation 3000, 4x/year

Recreational Equipment: Snow skis, boots, poles, water skis, life vests, rafts, saddles, tents, cookware and stove, water weights

Options for Independence
1095 N. Main
Logan, UT 84341

Phone: (801)753-5353

Contact: Kate Stephens

Programs: Canoeing, camping, hiking, rafting, dog sledding, alpine skiing

Utah Handicapped Skiers Association
P.O. Box 543
Roy, UT 84067-0543

Phone: (801)777-7029

Contact: Steve Peterson

Program: Alpine skiing

Vermont

Vermont Adaptive Ski and Sports Association
P.O. Box 261
Brownsville, VT 05037

Phones: (802)484-3525; (802)484-3925 Fax

Contact: Laura Farrell

Programs: Adaptive skiing, ice hockey, scuba diving, horseback riding, water-skiing, canoeing, swimming, cycling, camping, fishing, ice sledding, ice skating, sledge hockey and specialized camps

Major Events:

Event	Month
Ski Challenge	March
UT 100 Mile Endurance Run	July
50 Mile Bike or Run	October
Bike Across Vermont	September
Ski racing and Learn to Ski camps	Jan/Feb

Publication: Newsletter

Recreational Equipment: Mono-skis, bi-skis, sit-skis, dog cart, hand cycle, tandem, ice sledge, outriggers, walkers

VIRGINIA

Richmond Athletes With Disabilities (RAD) Sports

P.O. Box 311
Richmond, VA 23202

Phone: (804)747-7769

Contact: Suzie Groah, M.D.

Programs: Wheelchair tennis, karate, quad rugby, golf, snow-skiing, whitewater rafting, water-skiing, road racing, fishing, swimming, yoga, canoeing, fitness and bowling

Publication: RAD Newsletter

WASHINGTON

Disabled Sports USA Northwest ("Team USAble")

P.O. Box 4124
Bellingham, WA 98227

E-mail: dsusanw@dsusa.org

Phones: (360)676-0134 Voice/Fax; (360)733-6714 Voice Only

Contact: Doug Mackey

Web Site: http://www.dsusa.org/~dsusa/regions/nwreg/dsusanw/

Programs: Alpine skiing, soccer, kayaking, canoeing, camping, and educational programs

Major Events:

Event	Month
SkiAble Relay Race	April-March
Northwest Adaptive SkiFest	March
Ski to Sea Relay Race	May
Desolation/SoundKayak	
Camping Trip	September

Publications: Yearly magazine with circulation of 35,000, Quarterly newsletter

Recreational Equipment: Kayaks, canoes, bi-skis, mono-skis, outriggers, tethers, harness, reins, ski bibs, spreaders, ski-tip stabilizers

Footloose Sailing Association

2319 North 45th Street, #142
Seattle, WA 98103

E-Mail: bewing3@brigadoon.com

Phone: (206)382-2680

Contact: Bob Ewing

Web Site: http://www.dsusa.org/~dsusa/regions/nwreg/footloose/

Programs: Adapted sailing instruction, sailing regattas

Publications: Seasonal newsletter

Recreational Equipment: Adapted sailing equipment

A FINAL WORD

Parents and professionals should be aware of the enormous benefit of recreational activities in the role of social and personal confidence. Having a disability should not preclude a person's participating in activities that enhance enjoyment. It is always important in one's life to maintain a balance between work and play.

Recreation activities have probably been among the most visible areas of change for people with disabilities. There is hardly a sport activity that cannot include the participation of people with disabilities. For those who accept the challenge, nothing is off limits. Not everyone needs or wants to be a superstar, but everyone can attain a level of confidence in an activity that interests him or her. Parents must be supportive and encouraging to help their young people develop those interests and skills because, it is through the mastery of tasks that we all raise our level of self-esteem.

— REFERENCES —

Information Resources from NICHCY's Database

The following information was selected from numerous resources abstracted in NICHCY's database. The organizations listed are only a few of the many that provide various services and information about transition services. Additional publications and information are also available from the clearinghouses listed, and state and local education agencies. Please note that these addresses are subject to change without prior notice.

You may obtain copies of the laws discussed by writing to your Congressional Representative. Federal regulations are available by writing to: Superintendent of Documents, U.S. Government Printing Office, Washington, DC 20402. There is usually a charge for the documents. It is important that you include the title of the regulations.

Community Participation (Recreation and Leisure; Personal and Social Skills)

Directory for Disabled Travelers. Travelin' Talk, P.O. Box 3534, Clarksville, TN 37043, (615)552-6670.

Directory of Travel Agencies for the Disabled. 1996. Twin Peaks Press, P.O. Box 129, Vancouver, WA 98666, (800)637-2256.

Easy Access to National Parks: The Sierra Club Guide for the Disabled. 1992. Sierra Club Books, 100 Bush Street, # 1300, San Francisco, CA 94104, (415)921-1600.

Ford, A.; Davern, L.; Meyer, L.; Schnorr, R.; Black, J.; and Dempsey, P. 1989. "Recreation/Leisure." In A. Ford et al. (eds.), *The Syracuse Community-Referenced Curriculum Guide for Students With Moderate and Severe Disabilities* (pp. 63-75). Baltimore, MD: Paul H. Brookes. *[Available from Paul H. Brookes Publishing Co., P.O. Box 10624, Baltimore, MD 21285. Telephone: (800)638-3775.]*

Heal, L. W., Haney, J. I., and Amado, A. R. N. 1988. Integration of Individuals With Developmental Disabilities into the Community (2d ed.). Baltimore, MD: Paul H. Brookes.

Lakin, K. C., and Bruininks, R. H. (eds.). 1985. *Strategies for Achieving Community Integration of Developmentally Disabled Citizens.* Baltimore, MD: Paul H. Brookes.

Schleien, S. J., and Ray, M. T. 1988. *Community Recreation and Persons With Disabilities: Strategies for integration.* Baltimore, MD: Paul H. Brookes.

— ORGANIZATIONS —

American Camping Association. 1333 H Street NW, Washington, DC 20005, (202)326-6630.

Travel Buddy. P.O. Box 31146, Minneapolis, MN 54431, (612)881-5364.

US Department of the Interior. National Park, P.O. Box 37127, Washington, DC 20013.

— NEWSLETTERS —

Handicapped Travel Newsletter. P.O. Drawer 269, Athens, TX 75751, (903)677-1260.

Travelin' Talk Newsletter. P.O. Box 3534, Clarksville, TN 37043, (615)552-6670.

7

SOCIAL SKILLS

This chapter covers the following topics:

➤ The importance of developing social skills

➤ Acquiring social skills

➤ How families can help widen social experiences

➤ Avoiding social mistakes

➤ Fostering relationships: suggestions for young adults

THE IMPORTANCE OF DEVELOPING SOCIAL SKILLS

In the course of human development, there is probably no greater need than to attach, connect, or build gratifying human relationships. This human need is felt by all, whether disabled or not. It is vital that all children be given the opportunities to learn and practice the social skills considered appropriate by society. All children must learn how to conduct themselves in ways that allow them to develop relationships with other people. Parents must keep in mind that social skills pervade an individual's entire life, at home, in school, in the community, and at the workplace. An example of the significance of a deficit in social skills appears to be that a large percentage (nearly 90 percent) lost their jobs because of poor attitude and inappropriate behavior, rather than the lack of job skills.

Children with disabilities may find developing these skills more difficult than their peers without disabilities. As a result of a variety of learning or other cognitive disabilities, visual or hearing impairments, or a physical disability that limits their chances to socialize, children with disabilities may lack the exposure and experiences required to develop appropriate social skills. Most, however, are capable of learning these important "rules" (Duncan and Canty-Lemke 1986) and should be given opportunities to learn and practice them by teachers, parents and professionals.

119

ACQUIRING SOCIAL SKILLS

The development of social skills is a process that begins very early. We usually learn these skills from modeling significant individuals in our lives. The road to social skill development is filled with successes and mistakes. When the mistakes occur, parents usually provide us with a clear frame of reference so that we learn from our mistakes. The change in our behavior to more appropriate responses usually results from reward or punishment; both tend to shape our behavior. Rewards tell us what to do and punishments usually tell us what not to do.

A very important source of social skill modeling comes from friends. A child who is able to maintain a social awareness of other people's reactions will modify his or her behavior in accordance with the positive or negative responses from others. In the case of individuals with disabilities, however, this important feedback on performance may be denied (Duncan and Canty-Lemke 1986); some cannot learn the basics of social behavior. For others, social isolation plays a key role; how can a person get feedback on his or her social skills when little socializing takes place?

Socialization takes time; we are always fine-tuning these skills throughout our lives, as we are exposed to many new social situations at different developmental periods. The development of social skills relies on the ability of children and adults to

➤ observe the behavior of others as well as their own

➤ discuss possible behavioral options

➤ practice different skills in a variety of situations to see which ones result in positive feedback

➤ listen to constructive feedback from individuals whom they trust and respect

Individuals with disabilities may have difficulty with many of the skills mentioned above; as a result they may

➤ find it hard to take turns during conversations

➤ not be able to maintain eye contact

➤ experience difficulty being polite

➤ have problems maintaining attention

➤ not know how to repair misunderstandings

➤ not be able to find topics that are of mutual interest

➤ have problems distinguishing social cues (both verbal and nonverbal), for example, facial expressions or tone of voice

➤ find it hard to express what they mean if language problems exist

➤ have difficulty judging how close to stand to another person

To compound the problem, many individuals with these deficits are completely oblivious to their social clumsiness, and do not understand why their social lives are not fulfilling.

Appropriate behaviors can be taught to individuals with disabilities. Teaching can begin at home, with the parent playing a vital role in helping a child to socialize. Children should be included in family social activities where they have a part to play in the gatherings. They might

➤ greet people at the door

➤ take their coats

➤ show them where the chairs are

➤ offer them food

Remember, these early interactions lay the foundation for interactions in the future—many of which will take place outside the home—and in many cases, skills will have to be practiced one at a time.

To a certain degree, children may be protected and rescued from uncomfortable social situations by their parents and teachers throughout school. As most children grow older, however, they interact more and more with people in situations where direct supervision by concerned adults is not possible. Children can learn how to incorporate the early teachings so that they can make friends within their peer groups, learn more about socializing, and refine their social skills as they grow and mature. Friendships are important for all children to develop, because contact, understanding, and sharing with others are basic human needs. As children develop, the natural movement is away from parents and more toward a peer group attachment. Friends "serve central functions for children that parents do not, and they play a crucial role in shaping children's social skills and their sense of identity" (Rubin 1980, p. 12).

Unfortunately, many children with disabilities are socially isolated as a result of several factors.

➤ The presence of a disability may make peers shy away.

➤ Transportation to and from social events may be difficult.

➤ Special health care may be required, for example, a respirator.

➤ The individual with the disability may be reluctant to venture out socially.

Because a lack of appropriate social skills may contribute to a person's social isolation, the child is caught in a vicious cycle. The current educational trend toward inclusion is an attempt to remedy this social isolation and provide all students with positive social role models.

HOW PARENTS AND PROFESSIONALS CAN HELP WIDEN SOCIAL EXPERIENCES

Teaching social skills is one of the most difficult and frustrating experiences confronted by parents and professionals, particularly when the disability is characterized by concrete thinking. What makes it so difficult is that our social behavior varies in different contexts and children with disabilities may not be able to adjust as quickly as the situation requires.

Parents and professionals can provide a variety of experiences that widen their social circle in a number of ways.

➤ Emphasize good grooming and personal hygiene, and teach children the basics of self-care.

➤ Discuss and explore the characteristics of good friendships—what makes for good friendships, how friendships are formed and maintained, and some reasons why friendships may end.

➤ Model important social behaviors and then have the individual role-play any number of typical friendly interactions. Such interactions might include phone conversations, how to ask about another person's interests or describe one's own interests, how to invite a friend to the house, or how to suggest or share an activity with a friend.

➤ Help the child develop hobbies or pursue special interests.

➤ Encourage the child to pursue recreational and leisure activities in the community as mentioned in Chapter 6, Recreational and Leisure Options.

➤ Encourage the child to participate in extracurricular activities at school.

➤ Help the teenager find employment or volunteer positions in the community.

➤ Try not to overprotect. Although it is natural to want to shield a child from the possibility of failure, hurt feelings, and others' rejection, parents, particularly, must allow their children the opportunity to grow and stretch socially.

AVOIDING SOCIAL MISTAKES

Many individuals with disabilities need special help to avoid two types of social mistakes. The first includes those that occur when the person with a disability treats an acquaintance or a total stranger as if he or she were a dear and trusted friend. Individuals with mental retardation are particularly vulnerable to making these kinds of mistakes—for example, hugging or kissing a stranger who comes to the family home.

The second error generally involves doing or saying something in public that society considers unacceptable in that context, such as touching one's genitals or undressing in plain view of others. Committing either type of error can put the person with a disability into a vulnerable position in terms of breaking the law or opening the door to sexual exploitation.

Keep the following in mind:

➤ Teach the distinction between public and private through modeling, explanation, and persistence.

➤ When a child commits public-private errors, such as touching his or her genitals, immediately and calmly say, "No, that's private. We don't touch ourselves in public." Then, if possible, allow the child to go to a private place.

➤ Provide a place of privacy for the child to go to. Not only does this allow the child to understand the difference between public and private but it acknowledges his or her right as an individual to have and enjoy time alone.

FOSTERING RELATIONSHIPS: SUGGESTIONS FOR YOUNG ADULTS

(*Note:* This particular section is addressed directly to the individual with a disability.)

You've probably been thinking about what it means to have an adult relationship. Some questions you may be asking yourself are:

➤ Will I ever have an adult relationship—a boyfriend or girlfriend, a lover, a spouse?

➤ How will I meet this person?

➤ What will I talk about?

➤ What will I say about my disability?

➤ Will my disability distract the other person from seeing me for the whole and unique person I am?

➤ What can I do to foster a relationship and help it grow into something strong and meaningful for me?

Here are some ideas about relationships, selfhood, disability, love, sexuality, friendship, patience, hope, and fulfillment.

➤ Don't ever believe that no one will love you because you have a disability. People with disabilities can both love and be loved. Relationships are based upon friendship, trust, laughter, and respect—all of which combine to spark and maintain the love you find in a relationship.

➤ Involve yourself in a variety of such activities as work, community projects, and recreation. These activities will give you the opportunity to meet people. They will also help you grow as a person and avoid boredom and loneliness.

➤ A relationship is fostered through being a good listener and companion, a person who genuinely cares about others. Build trust and respect between you and the other person. Share activities and ideas. Romance can grow out of such solid ground.

➤ Keep up on current events. Being able to discuss a variety of topics can help conversations flow.

➤ Be patient in your search for connection with others. Relationships take time to develop. They cannot be forced. Don't settle for the first person who expresses an interest in you as a woman or a man, unless you are also interested in that person!

➤ Be open about your disability. Communicate how your disability will affect, and might interfere with, specific aspects of everyday life. Bring it up yourself, as the other person is often uncomfortable with introducing the topic. The burden of a disability requires that you make other people comfortable with it. How you talk about your disability with openness and humor will set the tone for the relationship.

➤ Open and frank discussion between you and your partner is the key to solving whatever unique considerations your disability presents. Between loving and trusting partners, however, mutual pleasure and fulfillment are possible.

A FINAL WORD

I think that the harder someone tries to directly focus on finding social, romantic, or sexual partners, the more difficult it becomes. I would advise any disabled person to balance out their life and become actively involved in work, community projects, recreation, and other activities that involve platonic relationships. Then, make a conscious effort to become interested in the people you come in contact with. Opportunities for social contact will be a natural outgrowth of these activities. Concentrate on being a friend first. The romantic part will follow by itself. The same thing holds true whether you're disabled or not. (Lois, from Kroll and Klein 1992, p. 30)

— REFERENCES —

Arsenault, C.C. (1990). Let's get together: A Handbook in Support of Building Relationships Between Individuals With Developmental Disabilities and Their Community. Boulder, CO: Development Disabilities Center. (Available from Publications Department, Development Disabilities Center, 1343 Iris Avenue, Boulder, CO 80304-2612. Telephone: (303) 441-1090.)

Champagne, M., and Walker-Hirsch, L. 1988. *Circles I: Intimacy and Relationships*. Santa Barbara, CA: James Stanfield.

Collett-Klingenberg, L., and Chadsey-Rusch, J. 1990. "Using a Cognitive Process Approach to Teach Social Skills." In F. R. Rusch (ed.), *Research in Secondary Special Education and Transition Employment*. Champaign, IL: Transition Research Institute. [Available from Transition Research Institute, College of Education, University of Illinois at Urbana-Champaign, 61 Childrens Research Center, 51 Gerty Drive, Champaign, IL 61820. Telephone: (217)333-2325.]

Edwards, J. P., and Elkins, T. E. 1988. *Just Between Us: A Social Sexual Training Guide for Parents and Professionals Who Have Concerns for Persons With Retardation*. Portland, OR: Ednick.

Fullwood, D. 1990. *Chances and Choices: Making Integration Work*. Baltimore, MD: Paul H. Brookes.

Goldstein, A. P. 1988. *The Prepare Curriculum: Teaching Prosocial Competencies*. Champaign, IL: Research Press.

Griffiths, D. M.; Quinsey, V. L.; and Hingsburger, D. 1989. *Changing Inappropriate Sexual Behavior*. Baltimore: Paul H. Brookes.

Interstate Research Associates. December 1989. *Improving Social Skills: A Guide for Teenagers, Young Adults, and Parents*. McLean, VA: Author.

Interstate Research Associates. October 1989. *Teaching Social Skills to Elementary School-Age Children: A Parent's Guide*. McLean, VA: Author.

Kroll, K., and Klein, E. L. 1992. *Enabling Romance: A Guide to Love, Sex, and Relationships for the Disabled (and the People Who Care About Them)*. New York: Crown.

Lehr, S., and Taylor, S. J. 1987. *Teaching Social Skills to Youngsters With Disabilities: A Manual for Parents*. Boston: Federation for Children With Special Needs and the Center for Human Policy. [Contact Monographs Department, Federation for Children with Special Needs, 95 Berkeley Street, Suite 104, Boston, MA 02116. Telephone: (800)331-0688 (in MA); (617)482-2915.]

Lutfiyya, Z. M. April 1991. *Personal Relationships and Social Networks: Facilitating the Participation of Individuals With Disabilities in Community Life*. Syracuse, NY: The Center on Human Policy.

Mannix, D. 1993. *Social Skills Activities for Special Children.* West Nyack, NY: The Center for Applied Research in Education.

Matson, J. L., and Ollendick, T. H. 1988. *Enhancing Children's Social Skills: Assessment and Training.* New York: Pergamon. [Available from Pergamon, c/o MacMillan, Front and Brown Streets, Riverside, NJ 08075. Telephone: (800)257-5755.]

Mind Your Manners. 1991. Santa Barbara, CA: James Stanfield. (This six-part video program introduces students to proper social behavior necessary for success in everyday situations. The program includes an introduction to why manners are important and explores manners at home, table manners, manners at school, manners in public, and greetings and conversations.)

O'Connell, M. February 1988. *The Gift of Hospitality: Opening the Doors of Community Life to People With Disabilities.* Evanston, IL: Center for Urban Affairs and Policy Research. [Available from Publications Department, Center for Urban Affairs and Policy Research, Nortwestern University, 2040 Sheridan Road, Evanston, IL 60208. Telephone: (708)491-8712.]

O'Connell, M. August 1988. *Getting Connected: How to Find Out About Groups and Organizations in Your Neighborhood.* Evanston, IL: Center for Urban Affairs and Policy Research.

Osman, B. and Blinder, H. 1992. *No One to Play With—The Social Side of Learning Disabilities.* Novato, CA: Academic Therapy Publications.

Rubin, Z. 1980. *Children's Friendships.* Cambridge, MA: Harvard University Press.

Social Skills for Daily Living. 1988. AGS Publishers Publishers, Building, Circle Pines, MN 55014, (800)328-2560.

Socialization and Sex Education: The Life Horizons Curriculum Module. 1991. Santa Barbara, CA: James Stanfield. (This set of teaching instructions is designed for professionals who want to help their students understand themselves better socially, physically, and psychologically.)

TIPS. 1991. Santa Barbara, CA: James Stanfield. (This seven-part program gives students 150 tips for successful social interaction. The different parts are: getting along with others, getting to know others, getting along with adults, having friends, enjoying free time, living in the community, and being on the job. The program is available in slide or video format.)

Valenti-Hein, D., and Mueser, K. T. (1991). *The Dating Skills Program: Teaching Social-Sexual Skills to Adults With Mental Retardation.* Worthington, OH: International Diagnostic Services, Inc.

Walker, P.; Edinger, B.; Willis, C.; and Kenney, M. 1989. *Beyond the Classroom: Involving Students With Severe Disabilities in Extracurricular Activities.* Syracuse, NY: Center on Human Policy, Syracuse University. [Available from Center on Human Policy, School of Education, Syracuse University, 200 Huntington Hall, 2d Floor, Syracuse, NY 13244-2340. Telephone: (315)443-3851.]

Weiner, F. (ed.). 1986. *No Apologies.* New York: St. Martin's Press.

8

SEXUAL ISSUES

This chapter covers the following topics:

➢ Misconceptions about sexuality and disabilities

➢ What is sexuality

➢ Sexuality and development

➢ Sexuality education

➢ Teaching children and youth about sexuality

➢ Early signs of puberty

➢ How particular disabilities affect sexuality and sexuality education

Today, because of the work of advocates and people with disabilities over the past half-century, American society is acknowledging that people with disabilities have the same rights as other citizens to contribute to and benefit from our society. This includes the right to education, employment, self-determination, and independence. We are also coming to recognize—albeit more slowly—that persons with disabilities have the right to experience and fulfill an important aspect of their individuality, namely, their sexuality. As with all rights, this right brings with it responsibilities—not only for the person with disabilities but also for that individual's parents and caregivers. Adequately preparing an individual for the transition to adulthood, with its many choices and responsibilities, is certainly one of the greatest challenges that parents and others face.

MISCONCEPTIONS ABOUT SEXUALITY AND DISABILITY

The natural course of human development means that, at some point in time, children will assume responsibility for their own lives, including their bodies. A parent faces this inescapable fact with powerful and often conflicting emotions: pride, alarm, nostalgia, disquiet, outright trepidation, and the bittersweet realization that the child soon will not be a child anymore. The role that parents and professionals play in a child's social-sexual development is a unique and crucial one. Through daily words and actions, and through what they do not say or do, parents and caregivers teach children the fundamentals of life:

the meaning of love, human contact and interaction, friendship, fear, anger, laughter, kindness, self-assertiveness, and so on.

While a parent is expected to be a child's primary educator of values, morals, and sexuality, this may often not be the case. For many reasons, some personal and some societal, parents often find sexuality a difficult subject to approach. Discussing sexuality with one's child may make a parent uncomfortable, regardless of whether the child has a disability, and regardless of culture or educational background, religious affiliation, beliefs, or life experiences. For many people, the word *sexuality* conjures up many images, both good (joy, family, warmth, pleasure, love) and fearful (sexually transmitted diseases, exploitation, unwanted pregnancies). Anxieties and misgivings are often heightened for parents of children with disabilities.

Unfortunately, there are many misconceptions about the sexuality of children with disabilities. The most common myth is that children and youth with disabilities are asexual and consequently do not need education about their sexuality. The truth is that all children are social and sexual beings from the day they are born (Sugar 1990). They grow and become adolescents with physically maturing bodies and a host of emerging social and sexual feelings and needs; this is true for the vast majority of young people, including those with disabilities. Many people also think that individuals with disabilities will not marry or have children, so they have no need to learn about sexuality. This is not true either. With increased realization of their rights, and more independence and self-sufficiency, people with disabilities are choosing to marry or to become sexually involved. As a consequence of increased choice and wider opportunity, children and youth with disabilities do have a genuine need to learn about sexuality—what sexuality is, its meaning in adolescent and adult life, and the responsibilities that go along with exploring and experiencing one's own sexuality. They need information about values, morals, and the subtleties of friendship, dating, love, and intimacy. They also need to know how to protect themselves against unwanted pregnancies, sexually transmitted diseases, and sexual exploitation.

WHAT IS SEXUALITY?

According to the Sex Information and Education Council of the U.S. (SIECUS):

> Human sexuality encompasses the sexual knowledge, beliefs, attitudes, values, and behaviors of individuals. It deals with the anatomy, physiology, and biochemistry of the sexual response system; with roles, identity, and personality; with individual thoughts, feelings, behaviors, and relationships. It addresses ethical, spiritual, and moral concerns, and group and cultural variations. (Haffner 1990, p. 28)

How Sexuality Develops

An understanding of sexuality begins with looking at how the social and sexual self develops. These two facets of the total self must be examined in conjunction with one another, for sexuality is not something that develops in isolation from other aspects of identity (Edwards and Elkins 1988). Indeed, much of what is appropriate sexual behavior is appropriate social behavior and involves learning to behave in socially acceptable ways.

From the time we are born, we are sexual beings, deriving enormous satisfaction from our own bodies and from our interactions with others, particularly the warm embraces of our mothers and fathers. Most infants delight in being stroked, rocked, held, and touched. Research shows that the amount of intimate and loving care we receive as infants "is essential to the development of healthy human sexuality" (Gardner 1986, p. 45). The tenderness and love babies receive during this period contribute to their ability to trust and to eventually receive and display tenderness and affection.

We form many of our ideas about life, affection, and relationships from our early observations. These ideas may last a lifetime, influencing how we view ourselves and interact with others. Because children are great imitators of the behaviors they observe, the environment of the home forms the foundation for their reactions and expectations in social situations. Some homes are warm, and affection is freely expressed through hugs and kisses. In other homes, people are more formal, and family members may seldom touch. The amount of humor, conversation, and interaction between various family members also differs from home to home. Some families share their deep feelings, while others do not. Children observe and absorb these early lessons about human interaction, and much of their later behaviors and expectations may reflect what they have seen those closest to them say or do.

In the preschool and early school years, children continue to be curious about their bodies and the bodies of the opposite sex. They make many explorations, using all their senses. Friendships, playmates, games and activities are important during this period to the continuing development of the sense of self within a social sphere.

With puberty, which starts between the ages of 9 and 13, children begin to undergo great physical change brought about by changes in hormonal balance (Dacey 1986). Physical changes are usually accompanied by a heightened sexual drive and some emotional upheaval due to self-consciousness and uncertainty as to what all the changes mean. Before the changes actually begin, it is important that parents talk calmly with their children about what lies ahead. This is a most important time for youth; many are filled with extreme sensitivity, self-consciousness, and feelings of inadequacy regarding their physical and social selves. Their bodies are changing, sometimes daily, displaying concrete evidence of their femaleness or maleness.

During puberty, all children need help in maintaining a good self-image. Adolescence follows puberty and often brings with it conflicts between children and parents or caregivers; As humans advance into adolescence, physical changes are often matched by new cognitive abilities and a desire to achieve greater independence from the family unit and others in authority. The desire for independence generally manifests itself in a number of ways. One is that adolescents may want to dress according to their own tastes, sporting unconventional clothes and hairstyles that may annoy or alarm their parents. Another is that adolescents often begin to place great importance on having their own friends and ideas, sometimes purposefully different from what parents desire. The influence of peers in particular seems to threaten parental influence.

Both parents and adolescents may experience the strain of this period in physical and emotional development. A parent, on the one hand, may feel an intense need to protect the adolescent from engaging in behavior for which he or she is not cognitively or emotionally ready (Tharinger 1987). A parent may fear that the child will be hurt, or that deeply held cultural or religious values will be sacrificed. On the other side of the equation, young people may be primarily concerned with developing an identity separate from the parents and with experiencing their rapidly developing physical, emotional, and cognitive selves (Dacey 1986). All children follow this developmental pattern—whether they have a disability or not—some at a slower and perhaps less intense rate, but they all eventually grow up.

SEXUALITY EDUCATION

What does it mean to provide sexuality education to children and youth? What type of information is provided and why? What goals do parents, caregivers, and professionals have when they teach children and youth about human sexuality? Sexuality education should encompass many things. It should not just mean providing information about the basic facts of life, reproduction, and sexual intercourse. "Comprehensive sexuality education addresses the biological, sociocultural, psychological, and spiritual dimensions of sexuality" (Haffner 1990, p. 28). According to the Sex Information and Education Council of the U.S., comprehensive sexuality education should address

➢ facts, data, and information

➢ feelings, values, and attitudes

➢ the skills to communicate effectively and to make responsible decisions (Haffner 1990, p. 28)

This approach to providing sexuality education clearly addresses the many facets of human sexuality. Stated in broader terms, the goals of comprehensive sexuality education are as follows:

➢ **Provide information.** All people have the right to accurate information about human growth and development, human reproduction, anatomy, physiology, masturbation, family life, pregnancy, childbirth, parenthood, sexual response, sexual orientation, contraception, abortion, sexual abuse, HIV/AIDS, and other sexually transmitted diseases.

➢ **Develop values.** Sexuality education gives young people the opportunity to question, explore, and assess attitudes, values, and insights about human sexuality. The goals of this exploration are to help young people understand family, religious, and cultural values, develop their own values, increase their self-esteem, develop insights about relationships with members of both genders, and understand their responsibilities to others.

➢ **Develop interpersonal skills.** Sexuality education can help young people develop skills in communication, decision making, assertiveness, peer refusal skills, and the ability to create satisfying relationships.

➢ **Develop responsibility.** Providing sexuality education helps young people to develop their concept of responsibility and to exercise that responsibility in sexual relationships. This is achieved by providing information about and helping young people to consider abstinence, resist pressure to become prematurely involved in sexual relationships, properly use contraception and take other health measures to prevent sexually related medical problems (such as teenage pregnancy and sexually transmitted diseases), and to resist sexual exploitation or abuse (Haffner 1990, p. 4).

When one considers this list, it becomes clear that a great deal of information about sexuality, relationships, and the self must be communicated to children and youth. In addition to providing this information, parents and professionals must allow children and youth opportunities for discussion and observation, as well as to practice important skills such as decision making, assertiveness, and socializing. Sexuality education is not achieved in a series of lectures that take place when children are approaching or experiencing puberty; sexuality education is a lifelong process and should begin as early in a child's life as possible.

Providing comprehensive sexuality education to children and youth with disabilities is particularly important and challenging because of their unique needs. These individuals often have fewer opportunities to acquire information from their peers; have fewer chances to observe, develop, and practice appropriate social and sexual behavior; may have a reading level that limits their access to information; may require special materials that explain sexuality in ways they can understand; and may need more time and repetition in order to understand the concepts presented to them.

With opportunities to learn about and discuss the many dimensions of human sexuality, young people with disabilities can gain an understanding of the role that sexuality plays in all our lives, the social aspects to human sexuality, and values and attitudes about sexuality and social and sexual behavior. They also can learn valuable interpersonal skills and develop an awareness of their own responsibility for their bodies and their actions. Ultimately, all that they learn prepares them to assume the responsibilities of adulthood, living, working, and socializing in personally meaningful ways within the community.

Suggestions for Teaching Children and Youth About Sexuality

This section offers some practical suggestions on how to take an active role in teaching children and youth with disabilities about sexuality. The discussion is organized by age groupings and the specific types of sexuality training that can be provided to individuals as they grow and mature. Although physical development is not much delayed for most individuals with disabilities, a child may not show certain behaviors or growth at the times indicated below. Depending on the nature of the disability, emotional maturity may not develop in some adolescents at the same rate as physical maturity. This does not mean that physical development won't occur. It will. Parents can help children to cope with physical and emotional development by anticipating it and talking openly about sexuality and the values and choices surrounding sexual expression. This will help prepare children and youth with disabilities to deal with their feelings in a healthy and responsible manner. It's important to realize that discussing sexuality will not create sexual feelings in young people. Those feelings are already there, because sexuality is a part of each human being throughout the entire life cycle.

Basic sexual education occurs over a long period of time, from infancy through age 11. During this period some of the topics that have to be addressed include:

➤ the correct names for the body parts and their functions

➤ the similarities and differences between girls and boys

➤ the fundamentals of reproduction and pregnancy

➤ the qualities of good relationships (friendship, love, communication, respect)

➤ decision-making skills, and the fact that all decisions have consequences

➤ the beginnings of social responsibility, values, and morals

➤ the acknowledgment that masturbation can be pleasurable but should be done in private

➤ avoiding and reporting sexual exploitation

Also during the later part of this developmental age range, preteens are usually busy with social development. They are becoming more preoccupied with what their peers think of them and, for many, body image may become an issue. If we think of the emphasis placed on physical beauty within our society—"perfect bodies," exercise, sports, make-up—it is not difficult to imagine why many preteens with disabilities (and certainly teenagers) have trouble feeling good about their bodies. Those with disabilities affecting the body may be particularly vulnerable to low self-esteem.

There are a number of things parents and professionals can do to help children and youth with disabilities improve self-esteem with regard to body image.

➤ The first action parents and professionals can take is to listen to the child and to allow the freedom and space for feelings of sensitivity, inadequacy, or unhappiness to be expressed. Be careful not to wave aside a child's concerns, particularly as they relate to his or her disability. If the disability is one that can cause a child to have legitimate difficulties with body image, then you need to acknowledge that fact calmly and tactfully. The disability is there; you know it and the child knows it. Pretending otherwise will not help a child develop a balanced and realistic sense of self.

➤ Encourage children with disabilities to focus on and develop their strengths, not what they perceive as bad points about their physical appearance; this is called "refocusing" (Pope, McHale, and Craighead 1988). Many people have also helped a child with a disability improve negative body image by encouraging improvements that can be made through good grooming, diet, and exercise. While it's important not to teach conformity for its own sake, fashionable clothes can often help any child feel more confident about body image.

➤ One of the most important things that parents can do during their children's prepubescent years is to prepare them for the changes that their bodies will soon undergo. No female should have to experience her first menses without knowing what is going on in her body; similarly, boys should be told that nocturnal emissions (or "wet dreams," as they are sometimes called) are a normal part of their physical development. To have these experiences without any prior knowledge of them can be very upsetting to a young person, a trauma that can easily be avoided by timely discussions between parent and child. Tell your child that these experiences are a natural part of growing up. Above all, do so before they occur.

EARLY SIGNS OF PUBERTY

Early signs of puberty include a rapid growth spurt, developing breast buds in girls, and sometimes an increase in "acting out" and other emotional behaviors. Additional topics of importance to address with children approaching puberty are

➤ sexuality as part of the total self

➤ more information on reproduction and pregnancy

➤ the importance of values in decision making

➤ communication within the family unit about sexuality

➤ masturbation (*see* discussion that follows)

➤ abstinence from sexual intercourse

➤ avoiding and reporting sexual abuse

➤ sexually transmitted diseases, including HIV/AIDS

During this period of adolescence, it is important for parents to let their child assume greater responsibility in terms of decision making. It is also important that adolescents have privacy and, as they demonstrate trustworthiness, increasingly greater degrees of independence. For many teenagers, this is an active social time, with many school functions and outings with friends. Many teenagers are dating; statistics show that many become sexually involved. For youth with disabilities, there may be some restrictions in opportunities for socializing and in their degree of independence. For some, it may be necessary to continue to teach distinctions between public and private. Appropriate sexuality means taking responsibility and knowing that sexual matters have their time and place.

ISSUES TO ADDRESS WITH THE ADOLESCENT

Puberty and adolescence are usually marked by feelings of extreme sensitivity about the body. An adolescent's concerns over body image may become more extreme during this time. Let the adolescent voice these concerns, while you reinforce ideas you've introduced about refocusing, good grooming, diet, and exercise. Without dismissing the feelings as a "phase you are going through," try to help the adolescent understand that some of the feelings are a part of growing up. Parents may arrange for the youth to talk with the family doctor without the parent being present. If necessary, parents can also talk to the doctor in advance to be sure he or she will be clear about the adolescent's concerns. If, however, an individual remains deeply troubled or angry about body image after supportive discussion within the family unit, it may be helpful to engage the services of a professional counselor. Counseling can be a good outlet for intense feelings, and often counselors can make recommendations that are useful to young people in their journey toward adulthood.

One topic that many parents find embarrassing to talk about with their children is masturbation. They will probably notice an increase in self-pleasuring behavior at this point in their child's development (and often before), and may feel in conflict about what to do, because of personal beliefs. Beliefs about the acceptability of this behavior are changing, however, the medical community as well as many religious groups now recognize masturbation as normal and harmless.

Masturbation "can be a way of becoming more comfortable with and enjoying one's sexuality by getting to know and like one's body" (Sex Information and Education Council of the U.S. 1991, p. 3). Masturbation only becomes a problem when it is practiced in an inappropriate place or is accompanied by strong feelings of guilt or fear (Edwards and Elkins 1988). How can parents avoid teaching their children guilt over normal behavior—especially if they themselves are not convinced? First, they may wish to talk to a family doctor, school nurse, or clergy—and may be surprised to find that what they were taught as children is no longer being approached in the same way. In dealing with children, parents must recognize that they communicate a great deal through their actions and reactions; they have the power to teach children guilt and fear—or that there are appropriate and inappropriate places for this behavior.

The child must be taught that touching one's genitals in public is socially inappropriate and that such behavior is acceptable only when one is alone and in a private place. Starting from very early in the child's life, when a parent first notices such behavior, it is important to accept the behavior calmly. When young children touch themselves in public, it is usually possible to distract them. During adolescence (and sometimes before), masturbation generally becomes more than an infrequent behavior of childhood, and distracting the youth's attention will not work. Furthermore, it denies the real needs of the person, instead of helping him or her to meet those needs in acceptable ways (Edwards and Elkins 1988).

Among the many other topics that an adolescent will need to know about are

➤ health care, including health-promoting behaviors such as regular check-ups, and breast and testicular self-exam

➤ sexuality as part of the total self

➤ communication, dating, love, and intimacy

➤ the importance of values in guiding one's behavior

➤ how alcohol and drug use influence decision making

➤ sexual intercourse and other ways to express sexuality

➤ birth control and the responsibilities of child-bearing

➤ reproduction and pregnancy (more detailed information than has previously been presented)

➤ condoms and disease prevention

Depending on the nature of an individual's disability, parents may have to present information in very simple, concrete ways, or discuss the topics in conjunction with other issues. The parent's responses to a child's behavior will reflect. Remember, young people are receiving information from other sources as well; it may be essential to include the entire family in the resolve to be frank and forthright, for a lot of information comes from siblings. Children may feel more comfortable asking their brothers and sisters questions than directly asking parents.

Parents and professionals must encourage a child to be involved in activities with others that provide social outlets, such as going to the community recreation center on weekends, going to sports events or a movie, joining a club or group at school or in the community, or having a friend over after school. These interactions help build social skills, develop a social network for a child, and provide him or her with opportunities to channel sexual energies in healthy, socially acceptable directions (Murphy and Corte 1986).

HOW PARTICULAR DISABILITIES AFFECT SEXUALITY AND SEXUALITY EDUCATION

Tailoring the pace and presentation of information to the needs of each young person with disabilities is very important. Parents and professionals must take into consideration

➤ how the child's particular disability may affect his or her social-sexual development

➤ how the disability affects the child's ability to learn information about sexual issues

➤ what extra information may have to be provided to address a child's special needs

A FINAL WORD

Understanding how a particular disability affects social-sexual development, how it affects the learning process, and how it affects sexual expression can help parents and professionals effectively approach talking to and teaching children about sexuality.

A plethora of information is available with regard to sexuality education and specific disabilities. Explore the many different views, the information, and the techniques that are available for this sensitive issue.*

— REFERENCES —

Becker, E. F. 1991. *Love-Where to Find It: How to Keep It.* Accent Books and Products, P.O. Box 700, Bloomington, IL 61702, (800)787-8444.

Bielunis, P. 1995. *New Horizons in Sexuality.* Accent Books and Products, P.O. Box 700, Bloomington, IL 61702, (800)787-8444.

Bernstein, N. R. 1990. "Sexuality in Adolescent Retardates." In M. Sugar (ed.), *Atypical Adolescence and Sexuality* (pp. 44-56). New York: W. W. Norton.

Calderone, M. S., and Johnson, E. W. 1990. *The Family Book About Sexuality* (rev. ed.). New York: Harper Collins.

Dacey, J. S. 1986. *Adolescents Today, Third Edition.* Glenview, IL: Scott Foresman and Co. (Book is out of print but may be available in public libraries.)

Edwards, J. P., and Elkins, T. E. 1988. *Just Between Us: A Social-Sexual Training Guide for Parents and Professionals Who Have Concerns for Persons With Retardation.* Portland, OR: Ednick.

Evans, J. W., and Evans, M. L. 1990. "Sensory Disability and Adolescent Sexuality." In M. Sugar (ed.), *Atypical Adolescence and Sexuality* (pp. 57-86). New York: W. W. Norton.

Gardner, N. E. S. 1986. *Sexuality.* In Summers, J. A. (ed.) *The Right to Grow Up: An Introduction to Adults With Developmental Disabilities* (pp. 45-66). Baltimore, MD: Paul H. Brooks. (Book is out of print but may be available in public libraries.)

Garee, B. and Cheever, R. 1991. (ed.). *Marriage and Disability.* Accent Books and Products, P.O. Box 700, Bloomington, IL 61702, (800)787-8444.

Gordon, S., and Gordon, J. 1989. *Raising a Child Conservatively in a Sexually Permissive World* (rev. ed.). New York: Simon and Schuster.

Greydamus, D. E.; Gunther, M. S.; Demarest, D. S.; and Sears, J. M. 1990. "Sexuality and the Chronically Ill Adolescent." In M. Haffner, D. W. March 1990. *Sex Education 2000: A Call to Action.* New York: Sex Information and Education Council of the U.S.

Johnson, E. W. 1989. *Love, Sex, and Growing Up.* New York: Bantam. (This book is written for pre-teens.)

Kroll, K., and Klein, E. 1992. *Enabling Romance: A Guide to Love, Sex, and Relationships for Disabled People (and the People Who Care About Them).* New York: Crown.

Lindemann, J. 1990. *SAFE: An HIV/AIDS Curriculum for Individuals With MR/DD.* Portland, OR: Oregon Health Sciences University.

---

*Adapted from the NICHY article entitled *Sexuality Education for Children and Youth.*

Mauro, R. *Finding Love and Intimacy*. 1994. Accent Books and Products, P.O. Box 700, Bloomington, IL 61702, (800)787-8444.

Murphy, L. and Corte, S. D. 1986. *Sex Education for the Special Parent/Special Child*. 2(2), 1-5.

Monat-Haller, R. K. 1992. *Understanding and Expressing Sexuality: Responsible Choices for Individuals With Developmental Disabilities*. Baltimore, MD: Paul H. Brookes.

National Guidelines Task Force. 1991. *Guidelines for Comprehensive Sexuality Education: Kindergarten-12th Grade*. New York: Sex Information and Education Council of the U.S. SIECUS position statements 1991.

Pueschel, S. M. 1988. *The Young Person With Down Syndrome: Transition From Adolescence to Adulthood*. Baltimore, MD: Paul H. Brookes.

Pope, A. W., McHale, S. M. and Craighead, W. E. 1988. *Self-Esteem Enhancement With Children and Adolescents*. NY: Pergamon.

Pueschel, S. M. (ed.). 1990. *Parent's Guide to Down Syndrome: Toward a Brighter Future*. Baltimore, MD: Paul H. Brookes.

Schwab, W. 1991. *Sexuality in Down Syndrome*. New York: National Down Syndrome Society. Sex education for persons with disabilities that hinder learning.

Siegel, P. C. 1991. *Changes in You for Boys*. Richmond, VA: Family Life Education Associates.

Siegel, P. C. 1991. *Changes in You for Girls*. Richmond, VA: Family Life Education Associates.

Sobsey, R. 1991. *Disability, Sexuality, and Abuse: Annotated Bibliography*. Baltimore, MD: Paul H. Brookes.

Sugar, M. (ed.). 1990. *Atypical Adolescence and Sexuality* (pp. 147-157). New York: W. W. Norton.

Tharinger, D. J. 1987. *Sexual Interests*. In A. Thomas and J. Grimes (eds.) *Children's Needs: Psychological Perspectives*. Washington, DC: National Association of School Psychologists.

Valenti-Hein, D., and Mueser, K. T. 1991. *The Dating Skills Program: Teaching Social-Sexual Skills to Adults With Mental Retardation*. Worthington, OH: International Diagnostic Services, Inc.

Weiner, F. (ed.). 1986. *No Apologies*. New York: St. Martin's Press.

— ORGANIZATIONS —

Coalition on Sexuality and Disability. 380 2nd Street, 4th Floor, New York, NY 10010, (212)242-3906.

SIECUS. 130 West 42nd Street, Suite 2500, New York, NY 10036, (212)819-9770.

9

COMMUNICATION AND ASSISTIVE TECHNOLOGY

This chapter covers the following topics:

➤ The definition of assistive technology

➤ Assistive technology devices

➤ Problem areas for the disabled in computer access

➤ Intended users of the technologies

➤ Current technologies

➤ Visual impairments and assistive technology

➤ Hearing impairments and assistive technology

➤ Mobility impairments and assistive technology

➤ Speech and language impairments and assistive technology

➤ Technology and assistive technology on the Internet

ASSISTIVE TECHNOLOGY DEFINED

Computers were designed to perform at maximum efficiency when used by the nondisabled, but almost all of us employ some type of adaptive technology when using the computer. Adaptive technology ranges from wearing eyeglasses or wrist supports, to simply adjusting the brightness of the screen display or the height and angle of the monitor. Broadly defined, assistive technology includes any device or piece of equipment that increases the independence of a person with disabilities. Assistive technology for the disabled, of course, is not new. For instance, the wheelchair has long been an indispensable assistive device for those with impaired mobility.

The distinction between adaptive technologies employed by the nondisabled and assistive technologies for the disabled blurs at times. Some of the assistive technologies designed for the disabled have proven so ergonomically sound that they have been incorporated as standard features. One such example is the placement of the keyboard on/off switch, which was designed so that people with motor impairments would not have to reach to the back of the machine to turn the power on and off.

Assistive technology has increased enormously the ability of those with disabilities to lead independent lives. Computer-based environmental control units allow users to turn on lights and appliances and open doors from a wheelchair. Augmentative communication devices enable those who cannot speak to voice thoughts and needs using touch- or light-activated keyboards coupled to synthetic speech systems. Screen reading programs for the blind, screen magnification systems for those with low vision, and special ability switches that permit the mobility impaired to use a computer are only a few examples of the technology by which the individuals gain access to the computer screen and keyboard.

WHAT ARE ASSISTIVE TECHNOLOGY DEVICES?

Any item, piece of equipment, or product system, whether acquired commercially or off the shelf, modified or customized, that increases, maintains, or improves functional capabilities of individuals with disabilities.

Assistive technology devices can be anything from a simple tool with no moving parts (e.g., a toothbrush with a built-up handle) to a sophisticated mechanical/electronic system (e.g., a robotic arm). Simple, mechanical devices are often referred to as "low tech" devices while computer-driven or complex assistive technology may be called "high tech." However, many people in the assistive technology field have argued that this complexity-based classification is not a useful one as there is no clear division between "simple" or low tech and "complex" or "high tech" devices. With the passage of the Rehabilitation Act Amendments of 1992 (PL 102-569), assistive technology devices and assistive technology services are now included as part of rehabilitation technology.

Source: Technology-Related Assistance for Individuals With Disabilities Act of 1988 (Public Law 100-407, August 19, 1988).

PROBLEM AREAS FOR THE DISABLED IN COMPUTER ACCESS

The user with disabilities wants access to the personal computer or network workstation for the same reasons as the nondisabled. Modifications and even alternatives to standard computer hardware and software are often necessary, however, to make the computer accessible for them. The standard personal computer system—disk drive, keyboard, mouse, monitor and screen—can present barriers to certain users with disabilities. Some common access problems are discussed here.

➤ **Disk drive.** Handling diskettes is impossible for some users because of lack of strength or dexterity. In addition, those with impaired mobility may not be able to turn the computer on or off if the power switch is located to the rear of the hardware, as is frequently the case.

➤ **Keyboard.** The standard QWERTY keyboard used on most personal computers is often inaccessible to people with impaired mobility or fine motor control. Many disabled users do not have the strength required to press the keys on a standard keyboard. Those with limited range of motion are not able to move their hands easily from the alphabetic keypad to the arrow keys, function keys, or number keypad. Other users with uncontrolled or involuntary hand movements make frequent typing errors by pressing the wrong key, or by pressing a key longer than normal, inadvertently activating the automatic key-repeat feature of many keyboards.

➢ **Mouse.** Using a standard two- or three-button mouse may not be possible for those with impaired vision, mobility, or motor control; successful use requires not only sufficient vision to follow the graphic representation of the mouse on-screen, but also adequate fine motor control and strength to activate and control the mouse. Manipulating text and graphic displays by clicking, pointing, and dragging with the mouse is an acquired computer skill for all users, and requires considerable practice before mastery. Use of a mouse also requires sufficient strength and motion in the shoulder and arm to position and manipulate the device on the desktop or mousepad.

➢ **Monitor and Screen.** The screen display is not accessible to blind users or those with low vision without magnification or text-to-speech conversion. On the other hand, the screen display is accessible to the deaf user, but requires modification so that audible error messages or "beeps" are converted to text that the deaf user can read.

INTENDED USERS OF THE TECHNOLOGIES

The five areas of human functioning are the ability to:

➢ see

➢ hear

➢ move about freely

➢ speak

➢ learn

These areas are so critically important that by almost any criteria, irreversible loss of any one of these abilities is disabling. Among college and university students, access to computers is most often compromised by impairments of vision, hearing, and mobility. For the disabled user with low vision, access to the computer requires one or more means of assistance: speech, large print, or Braille. The blind user employs speech, Braille, or a combination of the two. The hearing-impaired or deaf user usually adapts most easily to using the computer, since the standard medium of exchange between user and computer is visual. Often only minor modifications, such as an alternative to the audible warning beep, are needed for this user. Users with impaired mobility and motor disorders must be evaluated carefully so that their best remaining function is incorporated in the plan of access to the computer. The ability to stand and walk unassisted, the range of motion of the joints and spine, and any loss of muscle strength, motor control, or coordination are all considered when selecting the appropriate assistive technologies. A disabled user whose best voluntary, controlled movement is the raising of an eyebrow can be fitted with a switch to access the keyboard. Those with impaired mobility use alternative input devices such as joysticks, ability switches, and modified keyboards. Keyguards cut down on extra keystrokes, while software modifications deactivate the automatic keystroke repeat feature.

CURRENT TECHNOLOGIES

Visual Impairments

The technology available to computer users who are blind or have low vision is extensive. The choice of the appropriate technology depends on a number of factors. Among them are

➤   the cause of the visual loss

➤   the extent of loss of visual acuity

➤   the quality of peripheral vision

➤   any other physical or mental limitations that might affect use of a computer

Following are examples of assistive devices designed to help those with disabilities.

SPEECH AND BRAILLE

Software called outSPOKEN gives audio cues to on-screen visual images such as icons, windows, menus, and cursor location (the numeric keypad replaces the need for a mouse). The outSPOKEN program is compatible with the Macintosh operating system, so blind people can use a Macintosh just as sighted people do—in the office, at home, at school, anywhere.

Another program called Duxbury Braille Translator converts text to Braille and formats printing on a Braille embosser.

A synthetic speech system is composed of two parts; the synthesizer that does the speaking, and the screen access program that tells the synthesizer what to say. The synthesizers used with PCs are text-to-speech systems.

MAGNIFICATION

Several things can be done to enlarge the images on the screen. One solution, CloseView, is software that magnifies the screen image up to sixteen times its regular size. An enhanced version of this software, called inLARGE, is also available as a separate product from Berkeley Access.)

Other magnification solutions range from monitors that display images in multiple resolutions to magnification lenses that attach to the outside frame of the monitor. The individual may also want to consider using software that reads text aloud, so that instead of looking at the words on the computer, he or she can listen to them. Contact the companies listed in the References at the end of this chapter to learn more about their access products for people with vision impairments.

Persons with considerable vision may not need a screen magnification program. One alternative is a larger monitor, which can provide larger text and graphics while maintaining all the material on the screen. Also, in some applications, the size of the fonts can be increased considerably.

Permanent large-print key labels can be placed on each character, number, and punctuation mark of the standard keyboard. The visually impaired user may benefit from this adaptation, as do children.

Systems also exist that offer the ability to scan hard-copy text into a PC, which then magnifies it on the computer screen. These systems vary in price.

OPTICAL CHARACTER RECOGNITION SYSTEMS

Optical character recognition (OCR) technology offers blind and visually impaired persons the capacity to scan printed text and then speak it back in synthetic speech or save it to a computer. There are usually three essential elements to OCR technology—scanning, recognition, and reading text. The current generation of OCR systems provide very good accuracy and formatting capabilities at prices that are up to ten times lower than a few years ago.

Hearing Impairments

ALERTING DEVICES/SYSTEMS

The various alerting and alarm systems that signal deaf and hard-of-hearing people include

➤ security systems

➤ baby cry alarms

➤ smoke alarm systems

➤ doorbell alerting systems

➤ paging devices

➤ telephone signaling systems

➤ wake-up alarms

The signal may be visual (a flashing light); auditory (an increase in amplification; or vibrotactile (a vibrator). For instance, if an alarm clock is wired to a vibrotactile device under the bed pillow, the user is literally shaken awake. Auditory signals are sometimes used in conjunction with either visual or vibratory signals.

TELEPHONE AIDS

Amplification devices may include a specially wired telephone handset, with an amplification device, a portable amplifier that attaches to a phone. Such volume control handsets may provide up to 30 percent additional power for the listener who has a hearing loss. These devices may be used with or without an individual's hearing aid.

TTYs AND TDDs

Text telephones (TTY) and telecommunication devices (TDD) enable deaf and hard-of-hearing people to have conversations by typing messages that are sent through the telephone network. While these devices offer a major form of communication, they are rather slow devices, especially when compared with computers.

TELECAPTION ADAPTERS

These devices, sometimes referred to as television decoders, attach to the television and enable deaf and hard-of-hearing people to read captions on their television screens.

Mobility Impairments

Many adaptations are available to assist those with impaired mobility to use the computer. Although a standard keyboard and mouse are the input devices of choice for most people, other devices have been developed. Among the most frequently used are modified and alternate keyboards, ability switches, and headpointers and joysticks. Whatever the method, the computer treats the input from these methods as if it had been received through the standard keyboard. Descriptions of three of these follow.

MACINTOSH OPERATING SYSTEM

Keyboards. There are dozens of different kinds of keyboards for the Macintosh. Depending on personal abilities and preferences, any of a number of them may be appropriate. The right keyboard may be the kind that looks like a traditional keyboard, but has large, touch-sensitive keys to help make typing easier. Another has only seven keys and uses a typing technique called chording, originally designed for one-handed typists.

The Apple Adjustable Keyboard, another possibility, splits into two sections and conforms to the natural position of a person's arms to make typing comfortable. Other products include switch-operated, on-screen keyboards that allow an individual to type with almost any part of the body, and "smart" keyboards that permit customizing each key's position, size, and function.

Mouse Alternatives. The mouse's sensitivity can be fine-tuned to a degree by using software that comes with the Macintosh, but this kind of refinement may not adequately address the needs of the student with a mobility impairment. If that is the case, there are many from which to choose: head-controlled mice, trackballs (in effect a mouse turned upside down), joysticks, mice of different sizes and speeds, writing pads that function as mice, touch-sensitive screens that act as mice, and even remote-controlled mice. Another solution is Easy Access, a software program that comes with every Macintosh. The MouseKeys feature of Easy Access lets a person use the keyboard to control the cursor's movements. How do you determine which pointing device is the most appropriate? First, you must find out what's available; browse through a computer magazine devoted to Macintosh technology; there you'll find new and different pointing devices being advertised regularly.

Input Systems. With the right hardware and software, a Macintosh can become a powerful system for learning, working, and playing. Keyboards and mice are traditionally used to control personal computers. Although your child or student may not be able to use these devices, you can choose between a number of alternatives, including a voice recognition system that allows a person to control the computer by talking to it; an on-screen keyboard that facilitates typing without physically touching the keys; and a head-controlled keyboard or mouse that lets a person type using head movements.

PC OPERATING SYSTEM

Keystroke Modification and Mouse Emulation. Keystroke modification and mouse emulation programs provide various combinations of the following utilities:

➤ execution of multiple keystroke commands serially rather than simultaneously ("sticky-keys")

➤ modification of key-repeat function

➤ manipulation of mouse from keypad or keyboard

➤ alternatives to clicking and holding down mouse buttons

➤ provision of visible or audible feedback for keystrokes

[*Warning:* A problem may occur in accessing the pull-down menus in some programs when using a keystroke modification program. Most application programs require that you hold the Alt key at the same time you depress the pull-down menu's appropriate "hotkey" letter. With the "sticky-keys" function on, you can hit them sequentially instead—useful for a one-handed typist, or someone using a mouthstick or other device. If the program already requires that they be hit sequentially (e.g., WordPerfect 5.1 and earlier versions), however, the results are unpredictable!]

Consider the following modifications, also, to aid the person with mobility impairment:

➤ The keyguard is a lightweight overlay, often plastic, that fits over the regular keyboard; holes are punched out of the plastic so that each standard key can be pressed if chosen deliberately, either with the fingers or mouthstick. The keyguard cuts down on accidental keystrokes substantially.

➤ Software exists that will disable the automatic-repeat feature of most keys on the keyboard. Alternate keyboards come in many styles.

Speech, Language, and Learning Impairments

On-line computer instruction is a particularly good medium for intensive remedial training. The strengths of the computer in education include its capacity for constant, individual feedback to the student along with an unlimited ability to carry out drill and practice exercises until a subject is mastered. Computer packages have been designed to improve the speech and language capabilities of those with poor hearing and speech, and also to assist those with cognitive injuries or learning disabilities.

SPEECH COMMUNICATION

Most new computers have speech capability built in, which means that some notebook computers—in addition to doing everything that a regular computer does—can travel with you, helping you communicate with others. A portable computer is small and lightweight, so it can be carried around in a backpack or easily attached to a wheelchair, making it a versatile communication tool. Using "text-to-speech" software, the computer can create synthetic speech from typed-in words, allowing the computer to speak out loud any word or phrase. Some computers also have the ability to record and play back a person's own voice (somewhat like a tape recorder), which results in a very high-quality sound. Special software can help an individual manage speech so that he or she can access the appropriate words on demand. Libraries of pictures, symbols, and graphics are often used to build "picture communication boards," enabling speech samples to be selected quickly and easily.

Technology and Assistive Technology on the Internet

A wealth of resources is available today, thanks to the development of the Internet. This vast base of knowledge and information is a key resource for parents and professionals working with individuals with disabilities. Many valuable sites are available to educate, inform, and offer a wealth of guidance on the topic of assistive technology available to individuals with disabilities. The following is a partial list but contains many of the more complete sites on this topic.

Site: ABLEDATA
Location: gopher
Address: gopher//val dor.cc.buffalo.edu/11/.naric/.abledata

ABLEDATA is an extensive and dynamic database listing information on assistive technology available both commercially and noncommercially from domestic and international manufacturers and distributors. The field of assistive and rehabilitation technology holds much promise for people with disabilities. It is one of many keys that can unlock the doors to a life of greater independence for people with disabilities. However, assistive technology is nothing but another unfulfilled promise unless current, usable information on existing assistive devices and services is made available to any and all information seekers.

Site: Access First
Location: World Wide Web
Address: http://www.inforamp.net/~access/af1.htm

Access First provides the best in sales, training, and support for the sight-impaired, print-handicapped, and learning-disabled community. Our main services are those of consultants, instructors, and software developers. We have more than forty years' combined experience in the areas of high-technology sales and technical support, applications design, community networking, and funding resources. As end users ourselves, we understand and can address the special needs of the student and professional in the workplace.

Site: Adaptive Computing Technology Center
Location: World Wide Web
Address: http//www. missouri.edu/~ ccact

The mission of the Adaptive Computing Technology Center is to create access to technology in a manner that enhances integration. Adaptive technology makes input to the computer and feedback from the computer accessible to persons with disabilities. This can be achieved by combining adaptive devices with standard computer equipment.

Site: Alliance for Technology Access (ATA)
Location: World Wide Web
Address: http://marin.org/npo/ata

Providing access to empowering technology for children and adults with disabilities. The Alliance for Technology Access (ATA) helps to enhance the lives of people with disabilities through technology, by raising public awareness, implementing initiatives, and providing information and hands-on exploration at community resource centers.

Site: Apple Computer's Worldwide Disability Solutions Group
Location: World Wide Web
Address: http://www.apple.com/disability/welcome.html

This on-line version of the Mac Access Passport is a place where you can interactively learn about the kinds of products that make it possible to use a Macintosh computer if you have a disability. You can download the latest version of our product database, link directly with major organizations and manufacturers, find a collection of access software programs from Apple, and more.

Site: The Archimedes Project
Location: World Wide Web
Address: http://kanpai.stanford.edu/arch/arch.html

Project Archimedes seeks to promote equal access to information for individuals with disabilities by influencing the early design stages of tomorrow's computer-based technology.

Site: AZtech, Inc.
Location: World Wide Web
Address: http://cosmos.ot.buffalo.edu/aztech.html

AZtech, Inc. is a community-based enterprise, by and for persons with disabilities. The name AZtech, Inc. stands for A to Z assistive TECHnology. AZtech is operated by the Rehabilitation Engineering Research Center on Technology Evaluation and Transfer (RERC-TET). The RERC-TET is supported by a grant from the National Institute on Disability and Rehabilitation Research, U.S. Department of Education.

Site: Center for Excellence in Special Education Technology
Location: World Wide Web
Address: http://129.252.237.161/CFE.htm

The Center for Excellence in Special Education Technology (CFE/SET) works in conjunction with the ETC to demonstrate the use of technology for instruction of students with special needs. The CFE/SET serves as a facility for utilizing technology pertaining to special education and teacher preparation.

Site: The Center for Information Technology Accommodation (CITA)
Location: World Wide Web
Address: http://www.gsa.gov:80/coca

A clearinghouse of information about making information systems available to all users. Includes WWW design guidelines.

Site: DREAMMS for Kids
Location: World Wide Web
Address: http://users.aol.com/dreamms/main.html

DREAMMS for Kids, Inc. (Developmental Research for the Effective Advancement of Memory and Motor Skills) is a nonprofit parent and professional service agency that specializes in assistive technology-related research, development, and information dissemination. Founded in 1988 by the parents of a Down Syndrome child, DREAMMS is committed to facilitating the use of computers, assistive technologies, and quality instructional technologies for students and youth with special needs in schools, homes, and the community. Services include Newsletters, individually prepared Tech Paks, and special programs entitled Computers for Kids, and Tools for Transition.

Site: EASI: Equal Access to Software and Information
Location: World Wide Web
Address: http://www.isc.rit.edu/~easi

Site: EASI's (Easy Access to Software on the Internet) Seminars on Adaptive Computing
Location: gopher
Address: gopher://sjuvm.stjohns.edu/11/disabled/easi/easishop

Gopher server: EASI's Seminars on Adaptive Computing, EASI's Online Workshops on Adaptive Computing, Articles About EASI's Online Workshops on Adaptive Computing, Sample Syllabus of EASI's Online Workshops on Adaptive Computing.

Site: Fortec Institute of Electronics
Location: World Wide Web
Address: http://sun4.iaee.tuwien.ac.at/e359.3/abtb/abtb.html

This group was established to intensify and consolidate efforts related to research and development of new technical solutions for disabled and elderly persons.

Site: Information, Technology, and Disabilities Newsletter
Location: gopher
Address: gopher://sjuvm.stjohns.edu

Gopher server: Disability and Rehabilitation Resources; Education and Teaching Resources; Groups and Organizations.

Site: The International Society for Technology in Education
Location: World Wide Web
Address: http://isteonline.uoregon.edu

A nonprofit professional organization dedicated to the improvement of education through computer-based technology.

Site: MacAccess Passport Online
Location: World Wide Web
Address: http://www.apple.com/disability/Welcome.html

For more than a decade, Apple Computer, Inc. has been developing innovative products and programs designed to help individuals with disabilities lead more independent lives. One of these initiatives is MAP, the MacAccess Passport, a tool that helps consumers and professionals discover assistive technology solutions for Macintosh computers.

Site: National Center to Improve Practice
Location: World Wide Web
Address: http://www.edc.org/FSC/NCIP

The National Center to Improve Practice (NCIP) promotes the effective use of technology to enhance educational outcomes for students with sensory, cognitive, physical, and social/emotional disabilities.

Site: NCSA Accessibility Project
Location: World Wide Web
Address: http://bucky.aa.uic.edu

Welcome to the NCSA Mosaic Access Page, a resource for those interested in how people with disabilities can use the Internet and the World Wide Web.

Site: Plugged In
Location: World Wide Web
Address: http://www.pluggedin.org

Plugged In is a community access and training center for computers and the Internet in East Palo Alto, California. Our mission is to bring the educational and economic opportunities created by new technologies to low-income families in our community. We are open 7 days and 70 hours a week. We offer more than 30 classes to kids, teens, and adults and work in partnership with more than 10 community agencies.

Site: ProNotes Software
Location: World Wide Web
Address: http://www.pronotes.com

ProNotes is a leader in the field of speech recognition.

Site: Project Pursuit
Location: World Wide Web
Address: http://pursuit.rehab.uiuc.edu/pursuit/homepage.html

Here you will find a wealth of resources including: disability information; education accommodation resources; lessons on assistive technology and funding available for this technology; descriptions of careers in science, engineering, and mathematics; high school preparations for these careers; access to countless other information servers, and much more.

Site: Use of Hypertext in Education
Location: World Wide Web
Address: http://www.ncsa.uiuc.edu/SDG/IT94/Proceedings/Educ/rice.hyper-kids/Hyper.html

Special Education teachers need a wide variety of instructional strategies to meet the unique needs of their students. The uses of Mosaic as a learning tool, a tutorial, teacher-created games, whole-language exercises, and a library of supplemental curriculum materials are demonstrated. Specific examples of games, classroom exercises, and a step-by-step procedure for writing tutorials is presented. The conclusion is that Mosaic can be a valuable tool to improve teaching efficacy.

Site: WebABLE!
Location: World Wide Web
Address: http://www.webable.com

WebABLE! is the World Wide Web information repository for people with disabilities and accessibility solution providers. WebABLE! is dedicated to promoting the interests of adaptive, assistive, and access technology researchers, users, and manufacturers.

A FINAL WORD

No doubt the scope of assistive technology for the computer user will enlarge in the future. New opportunities for students in higher education will surely lead to increased assimilation into the work force upon graduation. Assistive technology for computer users supports the precept behind the Americans With Disabilities Act—that those who have disabilities should have equal access to all opportunities.

— REFERENCES —

Alliance for Technology Access. 1994. *Computer Resources for People With Disabilities: A Guide to Exploring Today's Assistive Technology.* Alameda, CA: Hunter House. [Available from Alliance for Technology Access, 2175 East Francisco Boulevard, Suite L, San Rafael, CA 94901. Telephone: (415)455-4575.]

Behrmann, M. M. November 1994. "Assistive Technology for Students With Mild Disabilities." *Intervention in School and Clinic* 30(2), 70-83.

Center for Developmental Disabilities (annual). *Assistive Technology Information and Program Referral: A Directory of Providers.* Columbia, SC: Author. [Available from Center for Developmental Disabilities, Department of Pediatrics, School of Medicine, University of South Carolina, Columbia, SC 29208. Telephone: (803)935-5270.]

Judge, G. 1992. *Parent Guidebook to Assistive Technology.* Augusta, ME: Maine CITE Project. [Available from Maine CITE Project, Education Network of Maine, 46 University Drive, Augusta, ME 04330. Telephone: (207)621-3195.]

MacKenzie, L. 1994. *The Complete Directory for People With Disabilities: Products, Resources, Books, and Services.* Lakeville, CT: Grey House. [Available from Grey House Publishing, Pocket Knife Square, Lakeville, CT 06039. Telephone: (800)562-2139; (203)435-0868.]

Menlove, M. Spring 1996. "A Checklist for Identifying Funding Sources for Assistive Technology." *TEACHING Exceptional Children* 28(3), 20-24.

Mueller, J. 1990. *The Workplace Workbook: An Illustrated Guide to Job Accommodation and Assistive Technology.* Chicago, IL: National Easter Seal Society. [Available from Publications Department, National Easter Seal Society, 230 West Monroe Street, Chicago, IL 60603. Telephone: (312)726-6200 (Voice); (312)726-4258 (TT).]

National Institute on Disability and Rehabilitation Research. 1995. *Directory of National Information Sources on Disabilities: 1994-95* (6th ed.). Washington, DC. [Available from NARIC, 8455 Colesville Road, Suite 935, Silver Spring, MD 20910. Telephone: (800)346-2742 (V/TT).]

Parette, Jr., H. P., Hourcade, J. J., and VanBierviet, A. Spring 1993. "Selection of Appropriate Technology for Children With Disabilities." *TEACHING Exceptional Children* 25(3), 18-23.

Parette, Jr., H. P., Hofmann, A., and VanBiervliet, A. Spring 1994. "The Professional's Role in Obtaining Funding for Assistive Technology for Infants and Toddlers With Disabilities." *TEACHING Exceptional Children* 26(3), 22-27.

Parette, Jr., H. P.; Murdick, N. L.; and Gartin, B. C. Winter 1996. "Mini-Grant to the Rescue! Using Community Resources to Obtain Assistive Technology Devices for Children With Disabilities." *TEACHING Exceptional Children* 28(2), 20-23.

Perry, M., and Garber, M. Winter 1993. "Technology Helps Parents Teach Their Children With Developmental Delays." *TEACHING Exceptional Children* 25(2), 8-11.

RESNA Technical Assistance Project. 1992. *Assistive Technology and the Individualized Education Program.* Arlington, VA. [Available from RESNA Technical Assistance Project, 1700 N. Moore Street, Suite 1540, Arlington, VA 22209. Telephone: (703)524-6686.]

Scherer, M. J. 1993. *Living in a State of Stuck: How Technology Impacts the Lives of People With Disabilities.* Cambridge, MA: Brookline. [Available from Brookline Books, P.O. Box 1047, Cambridge, MA 02238. Telephone: (800)666-2665.]

Storeygard, J.; Simmons, R.; Stumpf, M.; and Pavloglou, E. Fall 1993. "Making Computers Work for Students With Special Needs." *TEACHING Exceptional Children* 26(1), 22-24.

— MAGAZINES AND NEWSLETTERS —

Able. P.O. Box 395, Old Bethpage, NY 11804. Telephone: (516)939-2253. This monthly magazine is subtitled "The Newspaper Positively For, By, and About the Disabled." It focuses on resources, independent living, and daily life.

Accent on Living. Cheever Publishing, Inc., P.O. Box 700, Bloomington, IL 61702. Telephone: (309)378-2961. This quarterly magazine serves as a guide to services and information on daily living and equipment for persons with disabilities. Articles focus on personal experiences of persons with disabilities, ideas for making the activities of daily living easier, and new products and services.

Assistive Technology. RESNA Press, 1700 N. Moore Street, Suite 1540, Arlington, VA 22209. Telephone: (703)524-6686; (703)524 6639 (TT). This newsletter is published twice a year and provides assistive technology information to people with disabilities, including product comparisons, evaluations of new technologies, user experience and feedback, training, funding, and legislation.

Mainstream. 2973 Beech Street, San Diego, CA 92102. Telephone: (619)234-3138. Published ten times a year, this national magazine for people with disabilities features new products, technology, education, employment, housing, transportation, stories about people living independently, politics and advocacy, and travel and recreation.

Technology and Disability. Center for Assistive Technology, 515 Kimball Tower, SUNY at Buffalo, Buffalo, NY 14214. This is a quarterly peer-reviewed periodical that deals with the application of rehabilitative and assistive technology for persons with disabilities, particularly in the performance of major life functions: education, employment, and recreation.

Access Review Sensory Access Foundation. 385 Sherman Avenue, Suite 2, Palo Alto, CA 94306. Telephone: (415)329-0430. This is a consumer's guide to technology for people with vision impairments and includes profiles of new technology and resource listings.

— ORGANIZATIONS —

ABLEDATA Database Program. Macro International, 8455 Colesville Road, Suite 935, Silver Spring, MD 20910-3319. Telephone: (800)227-0216 (V/TT); (301)588-9284 (V/TT). The ABLEDATA project maintains a database on more than 20,000 assistive technology devices, both commercially produced and custom made. Requests for information are answered by NARIC (National Rehabilitation Information Center) information specialists or by ABLEDATA staff.

ACCENT on Information (AOI). P.O. Box 700, Bloomington, IL 61702. Telephone: (309)378-2961. ACCENT on Information is a computerized retrieval system containing information on products and devices that assist persons with physical disabilities. Also available is an AOL sister service called ACCENT Special Publications, which publishes and distributes a variety of books of interest to persons with disabilities, along with a Buyer's Guide that lists equipment devices to assist persons with disabilities in daily living activities.

Access/Abilities. P.O. Box 458, Mill Valley, CA 94942. Telephone: (415)388-3250. This organization provides information in many areas, including aids and appliances.

Alliance for Technology Access (ATA). 2175 East Francisco Boulevard, Suite L, San Rafael, CA 94901. Telephone: (415)455-4575. The Alliance for Technology Access (ATA) is a growing coalition of technology resource centers across the country that provide information, awareness, and training in the use of microcomputers to aid children and adults with disabilities. Callers are referred to the technology resource center nearest them.

American Foundation for Technology Assistance. Route 14, Box 230, Morganton, NC 28655 (704)438-9697. Serves disabled persons and organizations with special technology needs; provides funding.

Apple Computer, Inc. Worldwide Disability Solutions Group, Mail Stop 38DS, 1 Infinite Loop, Cupertino, CA 95014. Telephone: (408)974-7910 (Voice); (800)776-2333 (Voice); (408)974-7911 (TT). Apple's Worldwide Disability Solutions Group has developed a wide variety of materials in print, video, and electronic form to describe how personal computers can constructively influence the experience of having a disability. The database Macintosh Disability Resources lists adaptive devices and specialized software available to individuals with disabilities affecting physical mobility, cognition, speech, hearing, vision, and learning. The publication Independence Day describes strategies and solutions for tailoring personal computers to individual needs and objectives.

Assistive Technology Funding and Systems Change Project. United Cerebral Palsy Associations, 1660 L Street, N.W., Suite 700, Washington, DC 20036. Telephone: (800)827-0093 (Voice); (800)833-8272 (TT); (202)776-0406. This project provides information on where to look for funding for assistive technology devices and services, and how to advocate to obtain needed assistive technology.

DIRECT LINK for the disAbled, Inc. P.O. Box 1036, Solvang, CA 93464. Telephone: (805)688-1603 (Voice/TT). DIRECT LINK is a public benefit organization that provides information and resources for any disability-related question. The LINKUP database contains over 11,000 organizations, including device assessment centers and agencies offering direct services to persons with disabilities and their families.

IBM Corp. Special Needs Systems. 11400 Burnet Rd., Internal ZIP 9466, Austin, TX, 78758. Telephone: (800)426-4832 (Voice); (800)426-4833 (TT). IBM's Special Needs Systems provides information on available assistive technology. Information for persons with disabilities affecting learning, hearing, speech and language, mobility, and vision is provided, including vendor and support group names, addresses, and descriptions.

RESNA. 1700 N. Moore Street, Suite 1540, Arlington, VA 22209. Telephone: (703)524-6686. RESNA is currently operating a Technical Assistance Project, which can help callers identify the program in their state that is responsible for providing information, training, and technical assistance on assistive technology to individuals with disabilities.

Technical Aids and Assistance for the Disabled Center (TAAD). 1950 West Roosevelt Road, Chicago, IL 60608. Telephone: (312)421-3373 (Voice/TT); (800)346-2939 (Voice). TAAD is an organization created by the Committee on Personal Computers and the Handicapped (COPH-2) to provide options in using personal computer technology to persons with disabilities. The TADD Center provides advocacy and services with an emphasis on selection and application of microcomputers. TADD can also refer callers to their local resource center of the Alliance for Technology Access.

Trace Research and Development Center. S-151 Waisman Center, 1500 Highland Avenue, Madison, WI 53705. Telephone: (608)262-6966 (Voice); (608)263-5408 (TT). The center is primarily concerned with research and development in the areas of augmentative communication (conversation and writing) and computer access for persons with physical disabilities. The center does not manufacture or distribute equipment, but will make referrals to specific sources of information regarding equipment, software, service centers, related professionals, and other information networks. Publications include the Trace Resource Book, a reference volume listing and describing currently available products for communication, control, and computer access for persons with disabilities. All information is available in alternative formats for individuals unable to read or handle print materials.

— VISUAL IMPAIRMENTS AND ASSISTIVE TECHNOLOGY RESOURCES —

Speech and Braille

Berkeley Access. 2095 Rose Street, Berkeley, CA 94709, (510)540-5535; (510)540-5115 Fax; (510)540-0709 TTY. E-mail: access@berksys.com.

Outspoken. Duxbury Systems, Inc., 435 King Street, Littleton, MA 01460, (508)486-9766. Duxbury Braille Translator.

Telesensory. 455 North Bernardo Avenue, Mountain View, CA 94043, (800)537-3961. Braille Embossers.

Magnification

Berkeley Access. 2095 Rose Street, Berkeley, CA 94709, (510)540-5535; (510)540-5115 Fax; (510)540-0709 TTY. E-mail: access@berksys.com. inLARGE.

New Concepts Marketing. P.O. Box 261, Port Richey, FL 34673, (800)456-7097.

MAGNIFICATION LENSES

Sigma Designs, Inc. 47906 Bayside Parkway, Fremont, CA 94538, (510)770-0100. Multiple Resolution Monitors.

— HEARING IMPAIRMENTS AND ASSISTIVE TECHNOLOGY RESOURCES —

ADA Enterprises. 9 Abbey Lane, P.O. Box 191, Middleboro, MA 02346, Voice (800)545-4470.

American Loop Systems. 29 Silver Hill Road, Suite 100, Milford, MA 01757, Voice (800)438-5667; TTY/TDD (800)955-7204.

AMTEL. Eagle Point Industrial Center, 55 Pottstown Pike, Suite 800, Chester Springs, PA 19425, Voice/TTY (800)999-8903.

Compu-TTY, Inc./Krown Manufacturing. 3115 Lackland Rd., Forth Worth, TX 76116, Voice/TTY (800)366-9950.

Global Assistive Devices. 4950 North Dixie Highway #121, Fort Lauderdale, FL 33334, Voice (954)784-0035.

IBM Special Needs Systems. P.O. Box 1328, Boca Raton, FL 33429-1328, TTY (800)426-3383.

Lucent Technologies. 14250 Clayton Rd., Town and Country, MO 63017, Voice/TTY (800)233-1222.

Motorola Pagers. 1500 Gateway Blvd., Boynton Beach, FL 33426, Voice/TTY (800)548-9954.

Nationwide Flashing Signal Systems. (NFSS) 8120 Fenton Street, Silver Spring, MD 20910, TTY (301)589-6670; Voice (301)589-6671.

Phone TTY, Inc. 202 Lexington Avenue, Hackensack, NJ 07601, Voice (201)489-7889.

Siemans Hearing Instruments, Inc. 16 East Piper Lane, Prospect Heights, IL 60070, Voice (800)333-9083.

TeleSensory. 455 North Bernardo Avenue, P.O. Box 7455, Mountain View, CA 94309-7455, Voice (800)227-8418.

— MOBILITY IMPAIRMENTS AND ASSISTIVE TECHNOLOGY RESOURCES —

Keyboards

Don Johnston, Inc. P.O. Box 639, 1000 N. Rand, Wauconda, IL 60084, (800)999-4660. Ke:nx and Ke:nx On:Board.

IntelliTools. 5221 Central Avenue., Suite 205, Richmond, CA 94804, (800)899-6687. IntelliKeys.

In Touch Systems. 11 Westview Rd., Spring Valley, NY 10977, (800)332-6244; (914)354-7431. E-mail: 74425.1633@compuserve.com. Wand Keyboard.

TASH, Inc. Unit 1-91, Station St., Ajax, ON L1S 3H2 Canada, (905)686-4129. MacMini Keyboard.

Mice

Edmark. P.O. Box 3218, Redmond, WA 98073, (800)426-0856. Mac TouchWindow.

Kensington Microware. 2855 Campus Drive, Mateo, CA 94403, (800)535-4242. TurboMouse.

Logitech, Inc. 6565 Kaiser Drive, Fremont, CA 94555, (800)231-7717. MouseMan.

Input Devices

Articulate Systems, Inc. 600 West Cummings Park, Suite 4500, Woburn, MA 01801, (800)443-7077. PowerSecretary.

Madenta Communications. 9411A 20 Avenue, Edmonton, AB T6N 1E5 Canada, (800)661-8406. Doors.

Origin Instruments. 854 Greenview Drive, Grand Prairie, TX 75050, (214)606-8740. HeadMouse.

SPEECH AND LANGUAGE IMPAIRMENTS AND ASSISTIVE TECHNOLOGY RESOURCES

Don Johnston, Inc. P.O. Box 639, 1000 N. Rand, Wauconda, IL 60084, (800)999-4660. Talk:About and Write:OutLoud.

Mayer-Johnson Co. P.O. Box 1579, Solana Beach, CA 92075, (619)481-2489. Speaking Dynamically.

— PC FORMAT ASSISTIVE TECHNOLOGY RESOURCES —

AccessDOS (freeware). IBM Corporation, (800)426-7282. Canada: IBM Canada (800)465-1234. Provides "sticky-keys" feature, allows modification of key repeat function, provides audible feedback for keystrokes, allows mouse manipulation from the numeric keypad, allows some alternative input devices to emulate keyboard and mouse, functions through serial port. System requirements: 286SX, Microsoft compatible mouse, DOS 4.x. Even though one of the functions of AccessDOS is to allow a keypad to be used as a pointing device (mouse), you still must have a mouse and mouse drivers installed for it to work. If you happen on ver. 1.0, once loaded it will not allow you to enter Windows. This was corrected with ver. 1.1 (current version is 1.2). AccessDOS may be downloaded directly from IBM's Special Needs Web site: www.austin.ibm.com/pspinfo/snsaccesdos.html.

Al Squared. P.O. Box 669, Manchester, Ctr., VT 05255, (802)362-3612. ZoomText for DOS.

Artic Technologies. 55 Park Street, Troy, MI 48083, (810)588-7370. Magnum Deluxe.

Dragger (Windows). George Leotti, gleotti@omni.voicenet.com, available as Shareware. Permits dragging without holding down the left mouse button, simulates a double click by a single-click sequence. Registered version includes a dwell option. System requirements: 286SX, Windows 3.x.

DVORAK Keyboard layouts (freeware). Provides an alternative to the standard QWERTY keyboard layout, key locations modified to speed up typing and reduce fatigue, available in two-handed, right-hand and left-hand keyboard layouts (the two-handed DVORAK keyboard layout for Windows is included with Windows 3.11 and Windows 95). Unless you purchase a DVORAK keyboard, use of a DVORAK keyboard layout will cause the remapping of the keyboard keys. In other words, what the key front says will no longer match the character sent to your computer. This may be confusing to someone who has been taught to type using the standard QWERTY keyboard layout and may require the purchasing of labels for the keyboard keys to aid in typing. DVORAK keyboard labels, charts, and workbooks are available from Keytime (206)522-8973.

HandiSHIFT (DOS). Microsystems Software, (800)828-2600. Provides "sticky-keys" feature, allows disabling of key-repeat function, provides audible feedback for keystrokes, includes an onscreen "shift state" indicator. System requirements: 286SX, DOS 3.x, 1K RAM. Demo versions of Microsystems Software programs may be downloaded directly from their Web site: www.microsys.com/ftpintro.htm.

KeepKey (Windows). ACON ApS Software, available as Shareware. Provides "sticky-keys" feature, allows user to define which keys to hold, allows user to define amount of movement and period of time allowed when double-clicking, allows user to assign certain functions to mouse buttons or series of mouse clicks. System requirements: 286SX, DOS 4.x, Windows 3.x.

SoftSwitch (DOS and Windows). John Simmons. Allows all mouse functions (movement, clicking, dragging) to be controlled by one or more switches through a parallel, game, or serial port in Windows. A Microsoft mouse or special mouse adapter is required; a joystick can also be used to emulate a mouse. System requirements: 286SX, 24K RAM, free game, serial, or parallel port; joystick and/or switch adapters; VGA or SVGA recommended. SoftSwitch is actually a suite of access utilities that include a virtual keyboard, scanning, and Morse code entry.

SwitchMouse (Windows). OMS Development, (708)251-5787. Allows all mouse functions (movement, clicking, dragging) to be controlled by a single switch or, optionally, two switches; does not interfere with a regular mouse; does not require the presence of a physical mouse or mouse drivers; switch input may be through a serial, parallel, or game port via an available adapter; also allows a joystick to control the mouse. Requires: Adapter. Available by ftp from: ftp.net-com.com/pub/eb/ebohlman as swmouse.zip (Shareware).

Visionware. (800)828-1056. LP-DOS.

— ELECTRONIC RESOURCES — WEB SITES —

EASI. Equal Access to Software and Information is dedicated to collecting and disseminating up-to-date information about how to provide access for persons with disabilities to computing and information technology resources, and to assisting universities, colleges, schools, businesses and nonprofit organizations in making their information facilities accessible with the use of state-of-the-art adaptive computing technology. EASI is affiliated with the Association for Higher Education, with friends and volunteers in over forty countries. For more information about EASI: E-mail: *easi@educom.edu;* tel: (714)830-0301 (Pacific Standard Time Zone). EASI's World Wide Web page is at *http://www.rit.edu:80/~easi/.* Other helpful links include the *ADA and Disability Information* page and the Library of Congress page on the *National Library Service for the Blind and Physically Handicapped (NLS).*

Handicap News Archive. The archive is a comprehensive source of information for those with an interest in disabilities. Information on the ADA and related legislation is available, as are listings of national and local support groups, newsletters, and sources of state and federal assistance. Shareware for the disabled computer user can be downloaded. Anonymous ftp site: log on as anonymous to HANDICAP.SHEL.ISC-BR.COM or (129.189.4.184); or contact Bill McGarry by telephone: (203)337-1518; or by E-mail: wtm@bunker (Bitnet) or wtm@Shelden.Shel.isc-br.com (Internet).

10

POSTSECONDARY EDUCATIONAL OPTIONS

This chapter covers the following topics:

➤ Colleges and career education

➤ The law and its impact

➤ Disability-related support services

➤ Financial aid

➤ Issues to consider when looking into postsecondary education

➤ Checklist for assessing colleges for accessibility

➤ Accommodations for specific disabilities

➤ Distance learning

A number of years ago, students with disabilities had limited choices when it came to choosing a college or university that could provide accommodations. With the advent of the Americans With Disabilities Act, and the disabilities rights movement, accommodations for students with disabilities became commonplace. Now, one is able to apply to several different types of postsecondary educational institutions. The first type of school is the college or university that is specifically geared for a certain type of disability.

COLLEGES AND CAREER EDUCATION

Colleges offer an opportunity for individuals with disabilities to continue their education and earn tangible evidence of education such as a certificate or degree. Junior and community colleges offer a variety of courses that, upon successful completion of the prescribed courses, may lead to a certificate or associate's degree. Community colleges are publicly funded, have either no or low-cost tuition, and offer a wide range of programs, including vocational and occupational courses. They exist in or near many communities; generally the only admissions requirement is a high school diploma or its equivalent. Junior colleges are usually privately supported, and the majority provide programs in the liberal arts field. Four-year colleges and universities offer programs of study that lead to a bachelor's degree after successful completion of four years of prescribed course work.

THE LAW AND ITS IMPACT

In high school, the school district was responsible for providing any or all support services necessary for an individual with disabilities to participate in the educational process. The college or university does not have the same legal obligation. They are required by law to provide any reasonable accommodation that may be necessary for those with disabilities to have equal access to educational opportunities and services available to nondisabled peers, *if requested.*

Title II of the ADA covers state-funded schools such as universities, community colleges, and vocational schools. Title III covers private colleges and vocational schools. If a school receives federal dollars, regardless of whether it is private or public, it is also covered by the regulation of Section 504 of the Rehabilitation Act, requiring schools to make their programs accessible to qualified students with disabilities.

Under the provisions of Section 504, universities and colleges may not

➤ limit the number of students with disabilities

➤ make preadmission inquiries as to whether an applicant is disabled

➤ exclude a qualified student with a disability from a course of study

➤ discriminate in administering scholarships, fellowships and so on, on the basis of a disability

➤ establish rules or policies that may adversely affect students with disabilities

For college students with disabilities, academic adjustments may include adaptations in the way specific courses are conducted, the use of auxiliary equipment, and support staff and modifications in academic requirements. These modifications may include

➤ removing architectural barriers

➤ providing services such as readers, qualified interpreters, or note takers for deaf or hard-of-hearing students

➤ providing modifications, substitutions, or waivers of courses, major fields of study, or degree requirements on a case-by-case basis

➤ allowing extra time to complete exams

➤ using alternative forms for students to demonstrate course mastery

➤ permitting the use of computer software programs or other assistive technological devices to facilitate test-taking and study skills

DISABILITY-RELATED SUPPORT SERVICES

Many college campuses have an Office for Disabled Student Services or Office of Special Services. Others have designated the Dean of Students or some other administrator to provide this information and to coordinate necessary services and accommodations. At vocational schools or other training programs, the person responsible for disability services can usually provide this information.

There are also many publications that can tell more about the policies and programs that individual colleges and universities have established to address the needs of students with disabilities.

FINANCIAL AID

Another major question regarding postsecondary education or training opportunities is the availability of financial aid to help pay for tuition and living expenses. Obtaining financial aid can be a complex process, because laws are amended and eligibility requirements, policies, and disbursement of government funds change each year. Most money called "financial aid" is available to those studying only above the high school level (thus, financial aid is usually not available for adult education). The student must usually demonstrate the ability to benefit from the education or training in order to receive traditional financial aid.

The financial aid system is based upon a partnership between the student, parents, postsecondary educational institutions, state and federal government, and available private resources. For the student with a disability, the partnership may be extended to include a Vocational Rehabilitation Agency and the Social Security Administration. Such a partnership requires cooperation of all, and an understanding by each of their responsibilities within the financial aid process.

What Is Financial Aid?

Financial aid is a system of financial assistance to help individuals meet their educational expenses when their own resources are not sufficient. Three types of aid are available:

➤ **Grants**—gifts and scholarships that do not have to be repaid. (A list of available scholarship and financial aid resources can be found in Appendix F). This information on financial aid can usually be obtained through the high school guidance counselor.

➤ **Loans**—money borrowed to cover school cost that must be repaid (usually with interest) over a specific period of time (usually after the student has left school or graduated).

➤ **Work**—employment that enables a student to earn a portion of school costs.

The Federal Government contributes to all three types of student financial aid. These programs are explained in a booklet called *The Student Guide: Financial Aid From the U.S. Department of Education*. The programs described in the booklet are:

1. Federal Pell Grants

2. Federal Supplemental Educational Opportunity Grants (SEOG)

3. Federal Work-Study (FW-S)

4. Federal Perkins Loans

5. Federal Family Education Loans (FFEL) including:
   a. Federal Stafford Loans (subsidized and unsubsidized)
   b. Federal PLUS Loans

All of these programs are based upon financial need of the student and his or her family, except the unsubsidized Stafford and PLUS programs.

What Expenses Are Considered Disability Related?

In addition to the financial aid that one may receive for tuition, room, and board, there may be times when additional expenses, which may require further financial assistance, are incurred. These may include

➤ special equipment related to the disability and its maintenance

➤ expenses of services for personal use or study such as readers, interpreters, note takers, or personal care attendants

➤ transportation necessary to pursue an academic program, if regular transportation is not accessible

➤ medical expenses relating directly to the individual's disability that are not covered by insurance

Students should be sure to inform the aid administrator of disability-related expenses that may previously have been covered by the family budget. These may include food and veterinary bills for dog guides, batteries for hearing aids and a telecommunication device for the deaf (TDD) (now called a Typed Text QTT), or the cost of recruiting and training readers or personal care attendants. Often, leaving home necessitates the purchase of new or additional equipment that will allow the student to be independent at school. Students with disabilities should seek assistance from the Office of Disability Support Services and/or Financial Aid Office to determine disability-related expenses.

Regardless of whether the student is able to obtain any special equipment or services through the institution or elsewhere, it is still important to let the financial aid administrator know of any anticipated expenses. Such information is considered in the determination of the student's financial need, on which all aid decisions are based.

Vocational Rehabilitation and Financial Aid

The local Vocational Rehabilitation Agency has VR counselors who can help a person with a disability determine eligibility for assistance. The VR program is an eligibility program, rather than an entitlement program. To be eligible for services, an individual must have a disability that is a substantial handicap to employment and must have potential for employment as a result of rehabilitation services. The primary goal of a VR counselor is to make the client employable; therefore, the counselor will look closely at a student's educational plans in terms of job potential. While initial counseling and evaluation are open to all, the counselor may determine that a client is not eligible for other services based on state agency policies governing economic need, order of selection, and other policies of the agency.

Among the services that may be provided by VR Agencies to a student who is a client are

➤ tuition expenses

➤ treader services for persons who are blind or learning disabled

➤ interpreter services for people who are hearing impaired; individually prescribed aids and devices, which are authorized in advance in an Individualized Written Rehabilitation Program (I WRP) developed jointly by the client and the counselor

➤ ttelecommunications, sensory, and other technological aids and devices

➤ other goods and services, which help render an individual who is handicapped employable.

The above items may differ from state to state, or be subject to a test of a client's ability to pay or the use of available resources from another social service agency before a commitment of VR funds is made. To understand why there are differences among and between states' VR programs, one needs to know that the U.S. Department of Education, Rehabilitation Services Administration (RSA) administers the Rehabilitation Act, but each participating state administers its own program through the provisions of a state plan that has been developed under the guidelines of the Act and that has been approved by RSA.

ISSUES TO CONSIDER WHEN LOOKING INTO POSTSECONDARY EDUCATION

1. What are admission requirements?

2. What is the grade point average? ACT? SAT?

3. Are there special accommodations for individuals with disabilities to take entrance exams?

4. Are there special incentive programs?

5. Is there a disabled student service office on campus? How does one contact the office? Does it have a full-time person there or is it part time?

6. What kind of documentation is required to verify disabilities?

7. Is there a disabled student organization on campus? How to contact them.

8. How are the faculty informed of the necessary accommodations, if needed?

9. Is tutoring available? Is it individualized or group? Is there a cost involved?

10. Are note takers and readers available? Is there a cost involved? How are they trained?

11. Is it possible to arrange for tape recorder classes, computers, untimed testing, test readers?

12. Is it possible to relocate classes to more accessible sites?

13. What is the college's policy regarding course substitutes or waiver of curriculum requirements?

14. Are there developmental courses available? In what areas?

CHECKLIST FOR ASSESSING COLLEGES FOR ACCESSIBILITY

When looking for the right college, make sure to find what services are available through the Office of Services for Students With Disabilities on each campus. The office may be located in the Office of Student Affairs, or it may be listed independently. It is essential to obtain just as much information as possible about services for students with disabilities, and services that pertain to particular disabilities, before beginning classes.

The following are samples of questions parents and the student should consider asking a college representative:

➤ What services are offered (for example, readers, note takers, bus service)? Are there fees?

➤ What are the names of the director and staff people connected to these services? Is there a document that describes the various services?

➤ Can you introduce me to a student with my disability (or another disability) so I can learn from that person's experience? What arrangements do other students make in the same situation as mine?

➤ Who is available to assist in finding services on and off campus (for example, accessible apartments, restaurants, other)?

➤ Is there an office for the local Vocational Rehabilitation agency on campus? If not, where is it?

➤ What are the local organizations for individuals with disabilities such as mine? What services can I get through them (for example, Center for Independent Living, Personal Care Association listings)?

➤ How many students with disabilities attend this college until graduation? What history is there of my major department making accommodations?

➤ If accommodations are ever denied, what is the procedure to follow to contest the decision?

➤ How early does a qualified student have to start to make arrangements for putting textbooks on audiotape?

ACCOMMODATIONS FOR SPECIFIC DISABILITIES

The student should be sufficiently knowledgeable about his or her disability to address every concern, or potential concern, with those who will be offering services.

Visual Impairment

➤ Does the college offer training in finding one's way around campus? If not, how do I get the training; do you have a list of qualified instructors?

➤ Are readers paid or volunteer? Who pays? (Whether using a volunteer or paid reader, assess whether your needs are being provided for, and find a gracious but clear way to communicate to them if they are not. Ask the office: "Do you help locate readers? Do you have any suggestions for finding them?"

➤ Are large-print computer programs available to me? What other assistive technology is available? Where is the equipment located? Is there training to help me use the computers and accompanying software?

➤ What accommodations are there for taking exams? How and where are they usually taken? What responsibility do I have in the whole process? Can I work out my own arrangements if I so choose? Can I get the exams in an alternative medium, like large print, or Braille, or recorded?

➤ Is campus transportation accessible for me? Is there campus or city public transportation and is it accessible to me?

Hearing Impairment

➤ Will the Office of Services for Students With Disabilities arrange for interpreters? If so, how do I set that up with my class schedule? If not, will they provide assistance in locating them? Who pays?

➤ Are oral and sign language interpreters available?

➤ Are note takers available to record lectures for me, or do I have to find my own? Are they paid, and who pays? What is the procedure for payment?

➤ Does the campus have TDDs (Telecommunication Devices for the Deaf, sometimes called Text Telephones)?

➤ What are the provisions for safety in the dormitory in case of fire or other emergency? Do dormitory telephones have the capacity to have the volume turned up?

➤ Is captioning of speakers while they are speaking available?

➤ What amplification equipment is available? Can I borrow any of it for my own use?

Mobility Impairment

➤ Is there accessibility to buildings, classrooms, laboratories, and dormitories? How wide are the residence hall doorways and what is the accessibility of the bathrooms?

➤ Will there be any special problems or assistance with class registration?

➤ Will anyone assist me in arranging my schedule to include the required classes and still have enough time to go from one classroom in one building to another classroom in another building?

➤ Will I be able to reach and use all the equipment in the laboratory? If not, what arrangements must I make?

➤ If I need special adaptations to access computers, who will provide them?

➤ If I need adaptations to access the library catalog system, who will arrange for them?

➤ If the college has a large campus, is there accessible transportation, such as a lift-equipped van, to get from one area to another? Are there curb cuts and smooth sidewalks that I can manage with a wheelchair?

➤ Is driver evaluation and training available?

➤ If my wheelchair needs repair, can I get it done locally?

➤ Is there a dormitory or other residence that can assist people who require help with daily activities such as eating or dressing?

Learning Disability

➤ Remember that academic accommodations are based on documented type of learning disability and its severity. Your diagnostic papers must be written by a licensed medical or psychological examiner. Subtest standard scores must be listed as legal evidence of severity. Your school skill levels will not be sufficient, nor will an old Individualized Education Plan (IEP) contract.

➤ There is a high probability that whatever the accommodations recommended by the examiner, they will not exactly meet your needs in college. In some classes you will need no accommodations but in others you may face demands on your learning disability that no one thought of. For these reasons, it is imperative you understand your learning disability thoroughly enough to explain how it works to a person unfamiliar with learning disabilities.

➤ While the laws allow accommodations for diagnosed disabilities, the law does not entitle anyone to misrepresent his or her needs for the purpose of gaining advantage over nondisabled people. The law probably will not protect past accommodations in a different academic circumstance unless the need can be documented. If you should find yourself in a resistant environment within a college or university after you begin attending, you will need to have available your diagnostic papers and the current request for accommodations in order to be successful in advocating for your needs.

➤ Are academic accommodations uniform for everyone, or are they individualized according to the diagnostic papers (for example, note takers, extended test time)?

➤ Are the students with more severe learning disabilities expected to manage their own lives (for example, getting homework in on time, money management, school schedules)? Who is available to help when help is needed?

➤ How early does a qualified student have to start making arrangements for special exam conditions with the professor?

➤ If the learning disability causes more trouble than anticipated, can the course load be reworked?

➤ Are there counseling services available in case a student gets overwhelmed?

➤ May I have additional time for tests? Who arranges for the extra time? Do I do it, or does the professor, the Office of Services for Students With Disabilities, or the Dean?

➤ May I tape class lectures?

Chronic Health Condition

➤ What medical services are available locally? Are there rehabilitation units in local hospitals?

➤ How can I arrange my schedule to accommodate fatigue?

➤ Can arrangements be made for a personal care attendant if I need one?

The answers to these questions will give you an idea of where college is going to be easy and where it is going to be hard, in terms of accommodations. You may need to change some strategies, and you may need to push for support in areas where the services do not appear to meet your needs. The more you know in advance, the more effectively you will begin, and the more effective you will be in beginning this process.

DISTANCE LEARNING AND ADULTS WITH DISABILITIES

Off-campus education, or distance learning, is becoming increasingly popular in the adult or higher education community. To reach the growing number of nontraditional students (those who are other than 18-23 years old, embarking on postsecondary education directly from high school), some postsecondary institutions have become decentralized, having campuses in several locations. A result of decentralization is that education can be available to those unable to attend classes during the day or on a specific campus due to work, family, or other commitments.

Distance learning includes courses offered by educational institutions, businesses, or other entities away from the regular campus site by computer conferencing, cable TV, telephone conference calls, videocassettes, correspondence courses, or any combination of these. Some courses may be accessed by the student at home. Others may be offered at a public library, business headquarters, factory meeting room, or other community site. Such nontraditional settings, or "schools without walls" can provide nontraditional students with the flexibility they need in order to earn college degrees or obtain training for new careers. One result of the diverse demographic patterns emerging at this century's end is that a growing number of adults with disabilities are seeking educational and career opportunities.

Distance learning is an option for adults with disabilities who are unable to participate in regular campus classes. Distance learning programs constitute a part of the system of lifelong learning, which has been steadily expanding for many years. Change itself has become the rule, not the exception. Educational services are moving from the classroom at formal institutions of higher education to sites in businesses and community agencies, as well as being totally off-site, using electronic technology.

According to the Carnegie Commission on Higher Education (1985) over two-thirds of organized learning opportunities for adults are provided by a diverse array of schools and noncollegiate institutions. Not only are the higher education institutions changing, but so are the learners. Increasing numbers are attending on a part-time basis and view learning as a lifelong process.

Students with disabilities may participate in distance learning opportunities for various reasons. Some students may be unable to leave home or hospital. Others may participate in such programs to increase flexibility regarding scheduling and to increase control over the environment in which they perform their academic work. Since institutions offer different types of distance learning programs, students are advised to investigate the options.

Enrolling in a Distance Learning Program

SELECTING A PROGRAM

Distance learners are strongly advised to be sure the school is accredited. An accredited institution has earned recognition from an appropriate accrediting commission or association that determined the institution has met acceptable levels of educational quality. Be sure to check with the institution concerning its accreditation before enrolling in any program. In addition, all states have an agency overseeing higher education that can be consulted about accreditation.

When choosing a particular postsecondary institution, students should be aware of the importance of academic advising, and ask whether it will be offered through computer, telephone, or in person. Academic advisors for distance learners are usually available to discuss degree plans, course selection, prerequisite courses, course content, preparation of portfolios, graduate school, study skills, and other areas of concern. Students and advisors should be able to develop a degree program plan that outlines how the student will complete all or part of the remaining academic requirements. Most advisors realize that adults have numerous responsibilities, and they are usually ready to accommodate varied schedules and widely differing needs.

Access to the Student Services at the College

Many individuals with disabilities who access distance learning programs do not realize that they can use and benefit from the institution's student services, through the Dean of Students, Office of Special Services, or Office of Disability Support Services. To obtain such accommodations as print materials in alternate formats, extended time for completing the work, or use of an interpreter or note taker, students with disabilities must disclose and document their disability to the Disability Support Services Office. Students who are not able to visit the office are encouraged to fax or mail a letter of application, résumé, or other documentation to the office, so a career counselor can provide feedback. Students with disabilities have been able to perform practice interviews over the telephone with a career counselor. Students may also communicate with the campus financial aid office.

Students in distance learning programs should be able to access most of the programs in student services at community colleges and universities. Some distance learning programs operate from very small offices and are themselves not able to offer extensive student services, but will try to accommodate by referring the student to the services offered to on-campus students. To increase the success of students enrolled in distance learning programs, faculty and administrators are encouraged to be creative when seeking to provide academic and student services to students with disabilities.

As demand for education by persons with disabilities continues to grow, distance learning will be an important factor in facilitating access. Many adults with disabilities who have already successfully completed a traditional program can also participate in distance learning programs as a means of continuing lifelong learning.

A FINAL WORD

One of the major goals of the transition process is to facilitate an individual's arrival at his or her maximum potential. Within the last ten years, the opportunities for an individual with disabilities to achieve higher education have expanded greatly. Every year, more and more colleges and universities develop the necessary programs that allow these individuals to participate in this educational environment.

— REFERENCES —

A.D.D. and the College Student: Guide for High School and College Students With ADD. 1995. Magination Press.

Aune, E. and Ness, J. 1991. *Tools for Transition: Preparing Students With Learning Disabilities for Postsecondary Education.* Circle Pines, MN: AGS. [Available from American Guidance Service, Publishers Building, P.O. Box 99, Circle Pines, MN 55014-1796. Telephone: (800)328-2560. In MN, call (800)247 5053.]

Brinkerhoff, L; Shaw, S; and McQuire, J. *Promoting Postsecondary Education for Students With Learning Disabilities,* PRO-Ed Publishers, 8700 Shoal Creek Blvd., Austin, TX 78757. (512)451-3246.

Davie, A. R.; Hartman, R. C.; and Rendino, N. 1990. *On Campus With a Disability: Expanding Diversity at AASCU Institutions.* Washington, DC: American Association of State Colleges and Universities. [Available from AASCU Publications, One Dupont Circle, Suite 700, Washington, DC 20036. Telephone: (202)293-7070.]

Directory of College Facilities and Services for the Disabled (3d ed.). 1991. Phoenix, AR: Oryx Press. [Available from Oryx Press, 4041 North Central Avenue, Suite 700, Phoenix, AZ 85012-3397. Telephone: (800)279-6799.]

Lipkin, M. 1990. *The Schoolsearch Guide to Colleges With Programs Services for Students With Learning Disabilities.* Belmont, MA: Schoolsearch Press. [Available from Schoolsearch Press, 127 Marsh Street, Belmont, MA 02178. Telephone: (617)489-5785.]

Mangrum II, C. T., and Strichart, S. S. (eds.). 1992. *Peterson's Guide to Colleges With Programs for Learning Disabled Students.* Princeton, NJ: Peterson's Guides. [Available from Peterson's Guides, Department 5710, 166 Bunn Drive, P.O. Box 2123, Princeton, NJ 08540-0008.]

Michaels, C. (ed.). 1994. *Transition Strategies for Persons With Learning Disabilities.* Singular Publishing Co., San Diego., CA 92105. Telephone: (800)521-8545.

Schlachter, G. A., and Weber, R. D. 1992. *Financial Aid for the Disabled and Their Families: 1992-1994.* Redwood City, CA: Reference Service Press. [Available from Reference Service Press, 10 Twin Dolphin Drive, Suite B-308, Redwood City, CA 94065. Telephone: (415)594-0743.]

Tweed, P. K., and Tweed, J. C. 1989. *Colleges That Enable: A Guide to Support Services Offered to Physically Disabled Students on 40 U.S. Campuses.* New Wilmington, PA: Park Avenue Press. [Available from Jason Tweed, 855 N. Park Road, #H203, Wyomissing, PA 19610.]

— SELECTED DIRECTORIES —

Adult Learner's Guide to Alternative and External Degree Programs. 1993. American Council on Education. ORYX Press, 4041 N. Central Avenue, Phoenix, AZ 85012, (800)279-6799.

Directory of Distance Education Through Telecommunications. 1991. National University Continuing Education Association Division of Educational Telecommunications, One Dupont Circle, Suite 615, Washington, DC 20036, (202)659-3130.

The Distance Education Handbook: An Administrator's Guide for Rural and Remote Schools. ERIC/CRESS, P.O. Box 1348, Charleston, WV 25325, (800)624-9120.

Peterson's Guide to Independent Study. 1992. National University Continuing Education Association (NUCEA), Department 2341, P.O. Box 2123, Princeton, NJ 08543-2123, (800)338-3282.

— ORGANIZATIONS —

Center for Adult Learning and Educational Credentials. Programs on Noncollegiate Sponsored Instruction, American Council on Education, One Dupont Circle, Suite 250, Washington, DC 20036, (202)939-9490.

(The) Council for Adult and Experiential Learning. 223 West Jackson Blvd., Suite 510, Chicago, IL 60606, (312)922-5909.

Instructional Telecommunications Consortium, American Association for Community Colleges. One Dupont Circle, Suite 410, Washington, DC 20036, (202)728-0206.

National Home Study Council. 1601 18th Street NW, Washington, DC 20009, (202)234-5100.

Selected Institutions of Higher Education That Offer Distance Learning Programs

New York Institute of Technology/American Open University, Central Islip, NY 11722, (800)222-6948.

Queensborough Community College/CUNY External Education Program for the Homebound, 222-05 56th Avenue, Bayside, NY 11364, (718)631-6397.

Rio Salado Community College/Maricopa Community College District SUNDIAL Network, 640 North 1st Avenue, Phoenix, AZ 85003, (602)223-4000.

Rochester Institute of Technology Distance Learning Office, One Lomb Memorial Drive, P.O. Box 9887, Rochester, NY 14623, (716)475-5089.

(The) State University of New York/Regents College, 1450 Western College, Albany, NY 12203, (518)474-3703.

Thomas A. Edison State College Admissions Office, 101 W. State Street, CN 545, Trenton, NJ 08625, (609)984-1150.

(The) University of Maryland University College Admissions Office, University Blvd. at Adelphi Road, College Park, MD 20742, (800)777-6463.

11

ESTATE PLANNING
FOR PARENTS

This chapter covers the following topics:

➤ Overview of estate planning issues

➤ How the type of disability affects estate planning

➤ How to start planning your estate

➤ Things to take into consideration when planning your estate, and your child's estate

➤ How government benefits may be affected by estate planning

➤ Guardianship

➤ Conservatorship

➤ Types of guardianship and conservatorship

➤ Who can best serve as guardian/conservator

➤ Alternatives to guardianship and conservatorship
  – Representative payee
  – Power of attorney
  – Special needs trust
  – Joint bank account
  – Informal advocacy

➤ Consequences of not filing for guardianship or conservatorship

➤ Letter of intent

➤ Writing a will

➤ Establishing a will

PLANNING FOR YOUR CHILD WITH A DISABILITY

This chapter will focus on one very important and often complicated issue that parents confront when they have a son or daughter with any type of disability—how to plan their estate to best provide for the child's future security. Parents often may ask themselves:

➤ What will our son or daughter do when we are no longer here to provide help when it's needed?

➤ Where and how will our child live?

➤ Will he or she have enough income to sustain a decent quality of life?

Other questions parents may ask themselves focus on the estate planning process itself:

➤ How do I know that my estate plan is going to work?

➤ Do I have enough money to hire a lawyer and write a will?

➤ Do I even have anything to leave my children?

These are very difficult questions for parents to consider and difficult ones to answer. When a child has a disability—whether it is mild, moderate, or severe—parents have concerns about that child's future. The information provided in this chapter is relevant both to a family whose child is already independent or is expected to be so, and to one whose child will need moderate or extensive support or supervision throughout life.

As a parent, you may have a tentative plan in the back of your mind that one day, in the near or distant future, you will write a will that leaves your son or daughter with a disability sufficient resources to make his or her life secure. Many of you may have already written such a will, yet there are many things to know and consider when planning your estate.

For example, bequeathing a person with a disability any assets worth more than $2,000 may cause the person to become ineligible for government benefits such as SSI and Medicaid. For many individuals with disabilities, the loss of these benefits would be a devastating blow. In addition to the cash benefits and medical coverage that would be lost, the person would also lose any number of other government benefits that may be available to eligible persons with disabilities, such as supported employment and vocational rehabilitation services, group housing, job coaches, personal attendant care, and transportation assistance. Therefore, it is our hope that you, as a parent, will read and thoroughly consider the information presented in this chapter. The future security of your son or daughter with a disability may well depend upon the actions you take to establish an estate plan appropriate to your child's needs.

HOW THE TYPE OF DISABILITY AFFECTS ESTATE PLANNING

Disabilities, of course, can take many forms and have varying degrees of severity. The nature and severity of your child's disability will affect the nature of the estate plan that you, as a parent, develop.

Physical Disabilities or Health Impairments

Many individuals have physical disabilities or health impairments that do not affect their ability to manage financial or other affairs. If your son or daughter has such a condition, how to leave your estate depends on a number of factors. The primary factor will be whether your son or daughter receives (or may one day need to depend on) government benefits such as Supplemental Security Insurance (SSI), subsidized housing, personal attendant care, or Medicaid. If your child does receive (or may one day need to depend on) government benefits, then it is most important to create a special estate plan that does not negate his or her eligibility for those benefits. How to do this is discussed in some detail in this chapter

If your son or daughter with a physical disability or health impairment is not eligible for, or is not receiving, government benefits, you may be able to dispense with elaborate planning devices and merely leave your child money outright, as you would to any other individual. If you believe that the disability may reduce your son's or daughter's financial earning capability, you may want to take special care to leave a greater portion of your estate to this child. There are some exceptions to this simplified approach; for example, if you are concerned that a son or daughter with a disability may not responsibly handle an inheritance, then you can utilize a trust, just as you would for any other heir.

Another exception is if your child's disability or health impairment involves the possibility of deteriorating health and more involved health care needs in the future. While your son or daughter may be capable of earning money and managing an inheritance at present or in the immediate future, in twenty or thirty years' time, deteriorating health may make it difficult for him or her to maintain employment or pay for health care. Government benefits might then become critical to your child's security. Remember, benefits include much more than money; your child may also be eligible for valuable services such as health care, vocational rehabilitation, supported employment, subsidized housing, and personal attendant care. If, however, a child acquires too many assets through inheriting all or part of your estate, he or she may be ineligible for these benefits. Therefore, in order to protect your son's or daughter's eligibility for government benefits at some point in the future and to provide for his or her long-range needs, you may have to consider establishing a special estate plan.

Cognitive Disabilities or Mental Illness

If your son's or daughter's disability affects his or her mental capability, the need to create a special estate plan is more clear cut. Mental illness and cognitive disabilities often impair a person's ability to manage his or her own financial affairs while simultaneously increasing financial need. As a result, you must take care to ensure that there are assets available after your death to help your son or daughter, while also providing that the assets are protected from his or her inability to manage them. More information will be given later in this chapter.

HOW TO START PLANNING YOUR ESTATE

What to Consider

Parents who have a son or daughter with a disability should give careful consideration to developing an estate plan that provides for that person's future best interests. Here are some suggestions that can help you approach planning your estate.

First: Realistically assess your son's or daughter's disability and the prognosis for future development. If necessary, obtain a professional evaluation of your child's prospects, and capability to earn a living and to manage financial assets. If your son or daughter is already an adult, you should have a fairly clear understanding of his or her capabilities, but if your child is younger, it may be more difficult to predict

the future. In such cases, you should take a conservative view. It is better to antici-
pate all possibilities, good and bad, in such a way that you do not limit your loved
one's potential or set him or her up for unrealistic expectations. Remember, too, that
you can change your estate plan as more information about your child becomes
available.

Second: Carefully inventory your financial affairs. Estimate the size of your estate
(what you own) if you should die within the next year or the next ten years. Keep
in mind that the will you write governs your affairs at the time of your death, and
so it must be flexible enough to meet a variety of situations. Of course, you can
always write a new will, but you may never actually write it because of a hectic
schedule, procrastination, or oversight.

Third: Consider the living arrangements of your son or daughter with a disability.
Your child's living arrangements after your death are of paramount importance.
Every parent of an individual with a disability should give thought to the questions,
"If (my spouse and) I should die tomorrow, where would our child live? What are
the possibilities available to him or her?" The prospective living arrangements of
your son or daughter will have a tremendous impact on how your estate should be
distributed. Involved in answering the question of living arrangements is whether or
not your child will need a guardian or conservator to make decisions for him or her
after your death. If you conclude that a guardian or conservator is necessary, you
should be prepared to recommend a potential guardian or conservator in your will.

Fourth: Analyze the earning potential of your son or daughter; it is important to
determine how much your child can be expected to earn as a result of employment.
If he or she is currently employed, does this employment meet all of his or her living expenses, or only some? If your child is currently too young to be employed, you
will have to project into the future. In many cases, even if your son or daughter is
employed or expected to be employed at some point in the future, he or she will
require additional financial assistance.

Fifth: Consider which government benefits your son or daughter needs and is eligible to receive. Support for a person with a disability will usually come from state and
federal benefits. These might be actual case grants, such as social security or supplemental security income, or they might be in-kind support programs, such as subsidized housing or sheltered workshop employment.

As discussed in Chapter 13, Financial Concerns, government benefits can be divided into the following three categories.

1. Those categories that are unaffected by the financial resources of the beneficiary. For
    example, social security disability insurance (SSDI) beneficiaries receive their bene-
    fits without regard to financial need. Regardless of what a parent leaves to a son or
    daughter with a disability, the social security payments will still be forthcoming once
    the person has qualified for them.

2. Some government benefits, such as supplemental security income (SSI) and
    Medicaid, have financial eligibility requirements. If a person with a disability has too
    many assets or too much income, he or she is not eligible to receive some or all of
    these benefits. Someone who is eligible due to a lack of financial resources can
    become ineligible upon inheriting money, property, or other assets, leading to a

reduction or termination of the SSI benefits for that person. Therefore, if your son or daughter is receiving government benefits that have financial eligibility requirements, it is important to arrange your estate in a manner that will minimize his or her loss of benefits, especially SSI or Medicaid.

3. Government programs are available to individuals with disabilities where payment for services is determined according to the person's ability to pay. Many states will charge the individual with a disability for programmatic benefits if he or she has sufficient assets or income. The most striking is the charge that can be levied against residents of state mental institutions. For example, if a resident of a state hospital inherits a substantial sum of money, the state will begin charging the resident for the cost of residency in the state hospital and will continue to charge until all the money is exhausted, yet the services provided will be no different from the ones that he or she was previously receiving.

First, however, let us take a more in-depth look at the various parts that make up estate planning. These include the following:

➤ guardianship
➤ letter of intent/letter of instruction
➤ wills
➤ trusts

GUARDIANSHIP

Parents are the natural guardians of their children until the age of 18, when the power to make decisions on their behalf ends. A court must authorize any future guardianship powers once a person legally becomes an adult. In the past, most individuals with disabilities had public guardians or conservators. Although the Commissioner of Human Services was the technical guardian, the acting guardian or conservator was usually a staff member from the county social service department. In recent years, an effort has been made to recruit family members and other concerned individuals to assume the role of guardian or conservator.

The purpose of this section is to help family members and friends with the detailed decision-making process involved with seeking private guardianship or conservatorship. We will answer some of the common questions about what guardianship or conservatorship is and is not. We will also explore the decision-making process and legal obligations of being a guardian or conservator.

What Is Guardianship?

Guardianship is the result of a court hearing that establishes the need to appoint an individual (guardian) to assume substitute decision-making powers for another person (ward) who is not capable of exercising his or her rights due to incapacity or incompetence. The standard for determining incapacity generally requires that a person is functionally unable to care for self or property and cannot communicate decisions regarding care for self or property. This incapacity must be the result of a disorder or disability.

Guardianship is the most restrictive limitation on personal decision-making authority that a court can impose on a person. The ward automatically loses the right to vote, the right to choose where to live, the right to approve medical procedures, the right to enter contracts, and other essential decisions. The role of the guardian is to act in the best interests of the ward in making decisions regarding financial matters or personal needs that have been authorized by the court. The duties of a guardian are defined by law. Only a court can establish guardianship.

Conservatorship (Limited Guardianship)

Conservatorship is a less restrictive form of substitute decision making by a person (conservator), for another person (conservatee) that may include some, but not all, of the duties of guardianship. The conservatee does not automatically lose the right to vote because he or she is not considered incapacitated in all areas. Conservatorships can be tailored to include assistance with certain activities only. If the conservatee is capable of making some essential decisions, conservatorship is preferable to guardianship. A conservator's duties are established by the court based on law, and a formal hearing similar to a guardianship proceeding is required.

Types of Guardianship and Conservatorship

An individual can be appointed a guardian or conservator of the person, the estate, or both.

Guardian of the Person and Estate: Has the full scope of powers and duties concerning every major aspect of the ward's life.

Conservator of the Person and Estate: Has only some of the powers of the guardian.

Guardian of the Person: Makes decisions concerning the ward's place of living, care, comfort, maintenance, employment, training, personal effects, medical procedures, entering into contracts, and social/recreational needs.

Conservator of the Person: Has some of the powers of the guardian depending upon the person's needs.

Guardian of the Estate: Assumes responsibilities for taking control of the ward's property, preparing a written inventory, keeping adequate records, determining and collecting all income, paying debts from the ward's assets, paying taxes, and filing an annual written report to the court about the assets, receipts, and disbursements of the estate.

Conservator of the Estate: Assists the conservatee with those specific financial matters that the court has authorized.

Unless the person has substantial assets, it may not be necessary to seek guardianship or conservatorship of the estate since there are detailed accounting procedures required. If your family member does not have significant assets, consult the clerk of your local county probate court to see if the court will allow you to avoid seeking guardianship or conservatorship of the estate.

Who Can Best Serve as Guardian or Conservator?

A close relative or friend over the age of 18 is usually the best choice to be a guardian or conservator, as long as that person is willing and able to meet all the responsibilities. If a close relative or friend is not available, a concerned professional or representative from an organization offering guardianship or conservatorship services may be appropriate.

It is important to note that although parents may state in their will that they want a particular individual to serve as guardian or conservator after their death, this is not legally binding. That individual must still go to court and go through the same proceedings that the original guardian or conservator went through to obtain guardianship or conservatorship. Therefore, it is advisable to consider adding another family member or friend in the original petition to the court.

ALTERNATIVES TO GUARDIANSHIP AND CONSERVATORSHIP

Based on an assessment of the functional and decisional skill level of your family member, you may decide that one of the several alternatives to guardianship or conservatorship may be more appropriate. The alternatives that follow are considered "less restrictive" because they do not restrict an individual's rights as severely as guardianship or conservatorship.

Appointment of a Representative Payee

Individuals receiving Supplemental Security Income (SSI) or Social Security Disability Income (SSDI) may receive the benefit checks directly, or the checks can be sent to a representative payee who will assist the beneficiary with financial management and payment of obligations. A representative payee is appointed by the Social Security Administration, and is typically a parent or social worker. Court action is not needed to establish a representative payee, but regular reports must be submitted to the Social Security Administration detailing how the money was spent. A separate bank account must also be maintained for the beneficiary's money. Contact the Social Security Administration for further information on the appointment of a representative payee.

Power of Attorney

If the person is a competent adult, he or she may authorize, in a private written agreement, another individual to assume power of attorney. A power-of-attorney agreement authorizes a person to enter into legal agreements and manage financial affairs in the name of another person. The person given power of attorney does not have to be a lawyer; any competent person can play this role. A power-of-attorney agreement terminates upon the death of the principal, or if the principal is determined to be incompetent. You may want to consult with a lawyer before setting up a power-of-attorney agreement.

Special Needs Trust

The only reliable method of making sure that the inheritance actually reaches a person with a disability when he or she needs it is through the legal device known as a special needs trust (SNT). The SNT is developed to manage resources while maintaining the individual's eligibility for public assistance benefits.

This trust agreement for the benefit of a person with a disability allows for a fund to be created that will pay for items and services not covered by Medicaid and other governmental benefits. The trust should be set up by an attorney, and you may want to consult a financial planner for additional assistance. A trustee will be authorized to spend money on behalf of the individual with disabilities for supplemental purposes like recreational opportunities, vacations, personal items, Christmas and birthday gifts, and so forth. It is essential that you consult with an attorney so that all of the implications of any changes in the interpretation of the law are clearly understood and communicated to you.

The Social Security Administration has publications, entitled *Understanding SSI*, that discuss special needs trusts and should be carefully reviewed by you.

Joint Bank Account

An account set up by a bank allowing joint access to the account may allow you to supervise or assist your family member with finances. This type of informal assistance may be sufficient to monitor finances when minimal supervision is required.

Informal Advocacy

For families who choose not to go the route of guardianship, the other alternative is to seek out an informal advocate who will carry out the conditions as stated in your letter of intent. Be aware that you can appoint more than one advocate—each responsible for a different area of concern, for example, financial or legal needs, or a public agency to oversee your child's well-being. Relatives usually make the best advocates because of their special knowledge of the needs of the family member. A friend or professional may be able to assist on an occasional basis. Don't overlook the assistance that can be provided by natural support systems such as other family members, church communities, neighbors, social clubs, and so on. This informal advocate can assist your family member in meetings with case managers, social service providers, and individuals in the community, as well as in financial, social, employment, residence, or recreational issues that may be faced by your child.

CONSEQUENCES OF NOT FILING FOR GUARDIANSHIP OR CONSERVATORSHIP

Because the natural guardianship powers of parents ends when a son or daughter turns 18, parents may lose the right to access records and to make decisions unless authorization is obtained from the court. If guardianship or conservatorship is appropriate for your family member, failure to seek these powers may result in a loss of power to consent to ordinary or necessary medical care; loss of access to medical records; loss of authority to challenge school or residential facility programs; and other rights previously held. Your family member may also have trouble having an Individual Service Plan (ISP) developed. For an exact explanation of your rights under this section, contact a lawyer who specializes in the rights of the disabled.

LETTER OF INTENT*

What Is the Letter of Intent?

Simply put, the letter of intent is a document written by you (the parents or guardians) or other family members that describes your son's or daughter's history, his or her current status, and what you hope for your child in the future. You would be wise to write this letter today and add to it as the years go by, updating it when information about your son or daughter changes. To the maximum extent possible, it is also a good idea to involve your child in the writing of this letter, so that the letter truly represents your child.

---

*Adapted from the NICHCY article "Estate Planning for Persons With Disabilities" by Richard W. Fee.

The letter is then ready at any moment to be used by all the individuals who will be involved in caring for your son or daughter should you become ill or disabled yourself, or when you die. Even though the letter of intent is not a legal document, the courts and others can rely upon the letter for guidance in understanding your son or daughter, and following your wishes. In this way, you can continue to "speak out" on behalf of your son or daughter, providing insight and knowledge about his or her own best possible care.

What Happens Once the Letter of Intent Is Written?

Once you've written the letter of intent about your son or daughter, the first, most important thing to do is to let people know that there is a letter of intent available to be consulted. This might mean telling your other children (or relatives, neighbors, friends, workshop director, pastor, or case manager) why you have written the letter, what type of information it contains, and where the letter can be found. Put the letter in an easily accessible place, and make it clearly identifiable. Many parents also make copies of the letter and give it to their other children (or other concerned individuals).

Second, you should update the letter on a regular basis. Select one day out of each year (such as the last day of school or perhaps your son's or daughter's birthday) where you will review what you have written and add any new information of importance. Talk with your child each time and incorporate his or her ideas. After each addition, sign and date the letter. Should something change in your child's life, such as his or her caseworker or the medication he or she is taking, update the letter *immediately*. In conclusion—will your letter of intent overcome all of the obstacles to your son's or daughter's transition into someone else's care? No, of course not. The letter is of immediate usefulness, however, in coping with your son's or daughter's changed situation and, in the long term, will certainly help care providers understand and care for your child.

How to Involve Your Son or Daughter in Writing the Letter

How much you involve your son or daughter in writing the letter of intent will depend in large part upon his or her age and the nature and severity of the disability. It is only fitting that young adults and adult children be involved in planning their own lives to the maximum extent possible. Many individuals have disabilities that do not prevent their full or partial participation in the letter-writing process.

Before involving your child, however, you, as parents, might want to talk first between yourselves about the content of the letter and your ideas regarding your child's future. When you've agreed upon the basic information you feel should go in the letter, discuss each area with your son or daughter. Ask for your child's input about his or her favorite things to do, what type of education has been enjoyable and what might be pursued in the future, what type of employment he or she enjoys or envisions. Equally crucial to discuss are your child's future living arrangements: How does your child feel about the options you are considering listing in the letter of intent?

It's important for your child to realize that the letter is not a binding, legal document; it is written to give guidance, not edicts, to all those involved in caregiving in the future. If you fear that your child will be upset by talking about a future that does not involve you as parents, then you may wish to make the discussion simply about the future—what will happen when your child leaves high school or a postsecondary training program, what your child wants to be or do in the next ten years, where he or she wants to live. You may be surprised to find that discussing the future actually relieves your child. He or she may very well be worrying about what will happen when you are no longer there to provide whatever assistance is needed.

Involving your child in discussing and making decisions about the future may be more difficult if the individual has a disability that severely limits his or her ability to communicate or to judge between a variety of options. You, as parents, are probably the best judges of how much—and how—you can involve a son or daughter with a severe cognitive disability. For these children, the letter is especially critical; it will serve to communicate the vital information about themselves that they cannot.

What to Include in the Letter of Intent

While a letter of intent is not a legal document, it gives the future caregiver a very thorough specific description of your child, his or her need, and your wishes on your child's care in case you are no longer able. Keep in mind that the letters may vary in their content and scope; however, there are several general areas that should be addressed. These include:

➤ **Behavior Management:** What consistent approach has worked best in your absence?

➤ **Daily Living Skills:** Average daily schedule, activities.

➤ **Day Program or Work:** Present, past, and future.

➤ **Education:** You have a lifelong perspective of your son's or daughter's educational history and goals.

➤ **Employment:** What has your son or daughter enjoyed? Consider his or her goals, aspirations, and limitations.

➤ **Financial Issues:** Benefits, services, financial holdings, assets.

➤ **General Information on the Parents:** Vital statistics on the parents, that is, names, addresses, phone, social security numbers, blood type.

➤ **Leisure and Recreation:** Structured and unstructured activities, vacations, fitness programs.

➤ **Marital Status of the Individual With Disabilities:** If the student with disabilities is married, wife's or husband's name, address, phone.

➤ **Number of Dependents:** List the names, birthdates of dependent children.

➤ **Medical Care:** What has and has not worked with your son or daughter?

➤ **Medical History and Care:** Diagnosis, function, facilities, blood type, insurance, doctors' and dentists' names and addresses, mental status, other therapies, allergies, diseases, procedures, operations.

➤ **Other Relationships:** Friends, relatives with whom the individual has close relationships.

➤ **Religion:** Is there a special church, synagogue, or person your son or daughter relates to in the religious community? Faith, name of clergy, and participation.

➤ **Residence:** If something should happen to you tomorrow, where will your son or daughter live? What would be the best living arrangement? Does your child need adaptive devices?

➤ **Sibling Information:** Names, phone numbers, addresses, nature of relationship.

➤ **Social:** What activities make life meaningful for your son or daughter?

[*Note:* To see examples of letters of intent, refer to *Planning for the Future* (Russell et al. 1995).]

Additional Considerations

ADVOCATE/GUARDIAN

Who will look after, fight for, and be a friend to your son or daughter? (List three to four people.)

TRUSTEE(S)

Whom do you trust to manage your son's or daughter's supplementary funds? (List three to four people.)

For each applicable area mentioned in the letter of intent, consider your son's or daughter's future. List three to four options to guide future caregivers in decision making and interaction with your child. Draw upon what you know about your son or daughter, through observation and through discussion with your child, and share what you've learned!

The discussion here represents an overview of the possible areas that should be included in the letter of intent. Review the sources at the end of this chapter for examples and further information.

WRITING A WILL

All parents, but particularly parents of individuals with disabilities, should have a will. The object of the will is to ensure that all of the assets of the deceased parent are distributed according to his or her wishes. If at death you have no will, your property will be dispersed according to the law of the state in which you live at the time of your death. This law is called the state's *law of intestacy.* Although laws of intestacy vary from state to state, in general they provide that some percent of assets of the decedent passes to the surviving spouse and the rest is distributed to the children in equal shares. Writing a will is highly recommended, since the laws of intestacy are rarely the most desirable way to pass property to one's heirs.

Although it is theoretically possible for any individual to write a will on his or her own, it is unwise to do so. Because of the technical nature of wills, it is highly advisable to have a lawyer prepare one. Parents of individuals with disabilities particularly need legal advice, because they often have special planning concerns. If you do not have a lawyer, you *can* call the local bar association, which will provide you with the name of an attorney in your vicinity, but it is preferable to contact a local disabilities group, which may be able to put you in contact with an attorney familiar with estate planning for parents of persons with disabilities. Not all lawyers are familiar with the special needs associated with caring and providing for individuals with disabilities, and it is best to find one who has prepared estates for other parents who have sons or daughters with disabling conditions.

The cost of an attorney varies according to the attorney's standard fee and the complexities of the estate. The attorney can quote you a fee based upon an estimation of the work. If the fee quoted is beyond your immediate means, it may be possible to negotiate a lower fee or devise a payment plan with the attorney.

Remember, a will goes into effect only upon the death of the person who created it. Until death, the creator of the will can freely revoke, alter, or replace it.

ESTABLISHING A WILL

Four Possible Approaches

The following is a very brief summary of four options in establishing a will. A more thorough explanation of these options should be discussed with a lawyer who specializes in the disabled. Having decided what your son or daughter needs and what you own, you can now consider how best to assist him or her. There are four possible ways to do so.

First, you can disinherit your son or daughter with the disability. No state requires parents to leave money to their children, disabled or not. If your assets are relatively modest and your son's or daughter's needs relatively great, the best advice may be to disinherit your child by name and have him or her rely upon federal and state supports after your death. This may be the most prudent decision, particularly if you wish to help your other children.

Second, you can leave your son or daughter with a disability an outright gift. If your child with a disability is not receiving (and is not expected in the future to need) government benefits, this may prove to be a desirable course of action. Your son or daughter, if mentally competent, can hire whatever assistance he or she needs to help with managing the gift. If your child has a mental illness or cognitive disability, an outright gift is rarely a good idea, because he or she may not be able to handle the financial responsibilities.

Third, you can leave a morally obligated gift to another of your children. Morally obligated gifts are not a complete solution, since they may not be legally protected. They can be useful, however, for parents who have a modest amount of money and do not expect a lifetime of care for a son or daughter with a disability. If you merely want your other sons or daughters to use some of the inherited money to assist their sibling with special needs, this may be the best approach for you.

Fourth, you can establish a trust for your son or daughter with a disability. The point of a trust is to keep assets in a form that will be available to your son or daughter but that will not disqualify him or her for government benefits, if he or she might otherwise be eligible for them.

Worksheet for Costing Out Expenses of the Person With the Disability

Before contacting a lawyer, do some preliminary estimates on the expenses and monetary needs that your child may require. The following list was adapted from Richard Fee's NICHCY article, "Estate Planning for Persons With Disabilities":

INCOME

Government benefits   _____

Employment   _____

Other   _____

Total Monthly Income   _____

EXPENSES

Housing:

Rental   _____

Utilities   _____

Maintenance   _____

Cleaning items   _____

Laundry costs   _____

Other   _____

Care Assistance:

Live-in   _____

Respite   _____

Custodial   _____

Other   _____

Personal Needs:

Haircuts, beauty shop   _____

Telephone (basic, TT)   _____

Books, magazines, etc.   _____

Allowance   _____

Other   _____

Clothing   _____

Employment:

Transportation   _____

Workshop fees   _____

Attendant   _____

Training   _____

Other   _____

Education:

Transportation   _____

Fees   _____

Books, materials   _____

Other   _____

Special Equipment:

Environment control   _____

Elevator   _____

Repair of equipment   _____

Computer   _____

Audio books   _____

Ramp   _____

Guide dog   _____

Technical instruction   _____

Hearing aids/batteries   _____

Wheelchair   _____

Other   _____

Medical/Dental Care:

Medical/dental visits   _____

Therapy   _____

Nursing services   _____

Meals of attendants   _____

Drugs, medicine, etc.   _____

Transportation   _____

Other   _____

Food:

Meals, snacks—home _____

Outside of home _____

Special foods _____

Other _____

Social/Recreational:

Sports _____

Special Olympics _____

Spectator sports _____

Vacation _____

TV/VCR or rental _____

Camps _____

Transportation _____

Other _____

Automobile/Van:

Payments _____

Gas/oil/maintenance _____

Other _____

Insurance:

Medical/Dental _____

Burial _____

Automobile/van _____

Housing/rental _____

Other _____

Miscellaneous:

Total Expenses _____
  (*Subtract*)

Monthly Income
+ Government _____

Benefits
  (*Equals*)

Supplementary

Needs _____

A FINAL WORD AND DISCLAIMER

This chapter is intended to provide accurate information. It is not intended however, to render any legal, tax, accounting, or other professional advice or services. Use this chapter as a general guide only. This book contains information that was available only up to the time of printing, and laws do change with some frequency. Discuss your estate planning with a qualified attorney; don't rely solely on the information that you find here or in any other book.

— GLOSSARY —

adjudication—a legal procedure by which a court determines if an adult is mentally competent to make some or all decisions for self.

beneficiary—a person or legal entity (e.g., corporation, charitable institution) to whom property is given.

codicil—an addition to a last will and testament to change, explain, or add to its provisions.

consent—a legal concept referring to a person's action in approving a procedure in which he or she is involved, or that will affect him or her.

decedent—a deceased person.

defacto—based on particular circumstances (in fact); a legal concept referring to a situation in which a person acts in a manner that indicates his or her mental incompetence.

de jure—through the law; a legal concept referring to a court determination that an adult is mentally incompetent.

estate—(1) the property in which a living person has legal rights or interest; (2) the property left by a deceased person.

execution—(1) the fulfilling of any and all legal requirements necessary to make a legal document valid; (2) the enforcement of a legislative or judicial decree or judgment.

executor/executrix—a person named in the will to oversee the distribution of property listed in the will.

fiduciary—a person who handles another's money or property in a way that involves confidence and trust.

gift—the transfer of property from one person to another without any contract or consideration (exchange of money, goods, or services).

intestate—without last will and testament; estate of the person who dies is distributed under the *intestacy laws* of the decedent's state of residence.

whole-family approach—an approach to planning for the future that takes into consideration the needs and preferences of all family members who might be affected by decisions concerning a family member with a disability.

— REFERENCES —

Books

Berkobien, Richard. (newest guide.) *A Family Handbook on Future Planning.* [Available from ARC Publications Department, P.O. Box 1047, Arlington, TX 76004.] Topic: Resources for Families.

California State Council on Developmental Disabilities. 1992. *Parents' Handbook on Developmental Disabilities.* [Available from California State Council on Developmental Disabilities, 2000 "O" Street, Suite 100, Sacramento, CA 95814.] Topic: Developmental Disabilities.

Mount, Beth and Zwernik, Kay. 1988. *It's Never Too Early, It's Never Too Late.* [Available from Metropolitan Council, Mears Park Centre, 230 East Fifth Street, St. Paul, MN 55101.] Topic: Resources for Families.

Russell, L. M.; Grant, A.; Joseph, S.; and Fee, R. 1995. *Planning for the Future.* Evanston, IL: American Publishing Company. [Available from American Publishing Company, 814 South Blvd., Evanston, IL 60202. Telephone: (800)247-6553.] Topic: Providing a meaningful life for a child with a disability after your death.

Turnbull, H. R.; Turnbull, A. P.; Bronicki, G. J.; Summers, J. A.; and Roeder-Gordon, C. 1990. *Disability and the Family.* Disability and the Family: A Guide to Decisions for Adulthood. Baltimore, MD: Paul H. Brookes. [Available from Paul H. Brookes, P.O. Box 10624, Baltimore, MD 21285-0624, Telephone: (800)638-3775.] Topic: A guide to decisions for adulthood.

— ORGANIZATIONS —

Disabled and Alone/Life Services for the Handicapped, Inc. 352 Park Avenue South, New York, NY 10010, (212)532-6740; toll-free (800)995-0066. National organization that assists families in planning for the future.

National Institute on Life Planning for Persons With Disabilities. 1617 Lancaster Drive, Petaluma, CA 94954, (707)664-4235.

— ADDITIONAL RESOURCES ON TRUSTS AND WILLS —

Pamphlets

Assessing the Need for Guardianship or Conservatorship, ARC of Minnesota, 3225 Lyndale Ave. South, Minneapolis, MN 55408, (800)582-5256.

Disability Service Guide, 1995, Matrix, 320 Nova Albion Way, P.O. Box 6541, San Rafael, CA 94903-0541. Topic code: Resources for Families.

Guardianship, Conservatorship, Trusts, Wills, etc., (Sterling L. Ross, Jr., attorney, author), Protection and Advocacy, Inc., 100 Howe Avenue, Suite 185-N, Sacramento, CA 95825. Topic code: Wills, Trusts, and Estate Planning.

Social Security and Supplemental Security Income Benefits for Children With Disabilities, (a series of fact sheets), ARC, P.O. Box 1047, Arlington, TX 76004. Topic code: Resources for Families.

Magazines/Catalogs

The Communitas Communicator (quarterly), Communitas, Inc., Box 374, Manchester, CT 06040. Topic code: Community Integration.

Focus (quarterly), National Council on Disability—An Independent Federal Agency, 1331 F Street, NW, 10th Floor, Washington, DC 20004. Topic code: Resources for Families.

Futurity (monthly), Minnesota Governor's Planning Council on Developmental Disabilities, 300 Centennial Office Building, 658 Cedar Street, St. Paul, MN 55155. Topic code: Resources for Families.

NARIC Quarterly, A Newsletter of Disability and Rehabilitation Research and Resources (approx. quarterly), National Rehabilitation Research Center, 8455 Colesville Road, Suite 935, Silver Spring, MD 20910-3319. Topic: Resources for Families.

The Whole Community Catalogue: Welcoming People With Disabilities Into the Heart of Community Life, 1992, (David Wetherow, author), Communitas, Inc., Box 374, Manchester, CT 06040. Topic code: Community Integration.

Software

Will Maker, 1995, Nolo Press Self-Help Law Books and Software, 950 Parker Street, Berkeley, CA 94710. Telephone: (510)549-1976. Topic code: Wills, Trusts, and Estate Planning.

12

INSURANCE ISSUES
FOR PARENTS

This chapter covers the following topics:

➤ Insurance options

➤ HMOs (health management organizations)

➤ PPOs (preferred provider organizations)

➤ Indemnity plans

➤ Medicare

➤ Medicaid

➤ Medicaid waivers

Chronic illness, disability, or severe injury creates great stress for family and friends. The adjustment for a family with a child who has a severe or complex health issue can be very intense and taxing; the special needs of this child require a focus on many issues. Concerns surrounding the child's well-being, health, daily life, and constantly changing future expectations are magnified. As the health field changes and technology and terminology expand, parents must learn new skills and acquire a wide range of knowledge to ensure that a child's ongoing health needs are properly addressed.

With the expansion of technology and improved medical care also comes the burden of growing medical costs. As a result, parents of children with chronic disabilities have the added anxiety of finding the resources necessary for medical attention and recommended equipment.

A great deal of financial, social, and medical support is available within the community, state, or country, but it is up to the parent to wade through the vast amount of terminology, forms, agencies, issues, and so on to find the best direction for a particular child. The path to the correct resources will differ from family to family as a result of

➤ the family's personal financial situation

➤ the type of available health insurance

➤ the child's specific medical needs

➤ the state in which the family resides

➤ the family's understanding of its rights and responsibilities

EXPLORING INSURANCE OPTIONS

The importance of exploring all the available options and avenues of assistance cannot be stressed enough; being proactive in this area is essential. The first thing you need to know is how to locate general sources of medical, financial, and insurance assistance. Through these sources you will find the best quality health care at the least risk. Following this process can help you discover several options that may reduce your costs.

Medical care and insurance have gone through major changes in the last five years with the advent of HMOs, or health maintenance organizations. These organizations assist insurance companies by evaluating and authorizing appropriate medical care. The best available medical insurance policy for a child with disabilities may already have been determined by your company's insurance carrier. If you do not currently have a policy, or are considering changing your current policy, you will be confronted with many different options. Several individuals and agencies can be contacted for assistance in making this decision. They include

➤   the office of social services in the medical facility where your child is treated or cared for

➤   the primary care physician

➤   the agent or claims representative in the company with which you may have health insurance

➤   the billing department for a specific physician or medical facility

➤   your state department of health

When contacting these individuals or agencies, develop a script beforehand, and keep a piece of paper or notebook handy to take notes on each conversation. You will also have to keep track of offices to which you are referred, insurance policy details, and state support systems.

There are people who can help you identify resources in your own community and in your state, as well as help you learn the questions to ask. These people are the parents and care providers who have been there. They can empathize with the complexity of details—phone calls, correspondence, medical forms, financial forms, and lingering questions. It may be helpful to contact parent groups and disability organizations near you to ask for help in your research. Associations concerned with specific disabilities can provide helpful information. Even if there is not an association for your child's needs, another group whose members also have complex medical needs will have information on financing these needs.

When you contact these individuals or agencies, offer the following information so that they may give you the best options for your situation:

➤   the health care needs of your child

➤   your medical insurance situation

➤   your outstanding expenses

➤   what you need

KINDS OF INSURANCE POLICIES

Before choosing an insurance policy, contact your personnel department, insurance broker, or state department of insurance. You may want to consider one of the following three kinds of policies:

➢ a health maintenance organization (HMO)

➢ an indemnity plan

➢ a preferred provider organization (PPO)

Health maintenance organizations represent prepaid or "capitated" insurance plans in which individuals or their employers pay a fixed monthly fee for services, instead of a separate charge for each visit or service. The monthly fees remain the same, regardless of the types or levels of services provided. There is usually a small copayment required for approved doctor's visits. Services are provided by physicians employed by, or under contract with, the HMO. HMOs vary in design. Depending on the type of HMO, services may be provided in a central facility or in a physician's own office.

Indemnity health insurance plans are also called *fee-for-service*. These plans existed before the rise of HMOs. With indemnity plans, the individual pays a predetermined percentage of the cost of health care services, and the insurance company (or self-insured employer) pays the other percentage. For example, an individual might pay 20 percent for services and the insurance company 80 percent. The fees for services are defined by the providers and vary from physician to physician. Indemnity health plans offer individuals the freedom to choose their health care professionals.

Preferred provider organizations (PPOs) offer you or your employer discounted rates if you use doctors from a preselected group. If you use a physician outside the PPO plan, you must pay more for the medical care.

Calculated Decisions

Deciding between an HMO, PPO, or indemnity plan is usually based on personal preferences with respect to freedom of choice and one's ability to pay for that freedom. There are medical factors, however, that may influence an individual's informed decision. You may also want to consider the following by estimating the expected, predictable health care needs of each family member over the next year:

1. How many visits to the doctor are expected for such preventive services as childhood immunizations, mammograms, pap tests, or sigmoidoscopies?

2. Are you planning to start a family? Will the child be born in the current year or next?

3. Do you have a chronic condition, such as diabetes, that requires ongoing medication?

4. What is your philosophy about medical services and health care professionals? Do you tend to go to the doctor for minor problems that in most cases would clear up on their own? Do you practice medical self-care in attempts to avoid going to the physician?

5. What was the average cost for health care services for you and your family over the past two years?

Try to estimate the likelihood of unpredictable health care needs of each family member over the next year. Ask yourself the following questions:

1. How healthy have you and your family members been in the past?

2. Do you or a member of the family have a chronic condition that requires sporadic visits to a health care professional?

3. Do you smoke?

4. Do you consume more than a reasonable amount of alcohol, that is, according to state standards?

5. Are you sedentary or do you exercise regularly?

6. Are you in an occupation that can be hazardous to your health?

While answers to the above will not tell you which plan is best for you and your family, they can help you estimate your health care costs over the next year. Then, you can compare the estimated costs of the various plans to see which plan is likely to be the best for you.

MEDICARE

Born out of the 1960s, Medicare was a response to growing concerns about the high cost of medical care for older Americans. Since that time however, the program has expanded to include not only older Americans but millions of adults with disabilities. Unlike Medicaid (discussed later) which is based solely on financial need, the right to Medicare benefits is established primarily by payroll tax contributions. Medicare is a federal health care insurance program that provides some medical coverage to people over 65 and also to individuals with disabilities for a limited period of time. Medicare will help meet some bills for long-term care, but will not fund unlimited long-term care. To meet uncovered costs, you may need supplemental or "medigap" insurance policies. Medigap insurance is offered by private insurance companies, not the government. It is not the same as Medicare or Medicaid. These policies are designed to pay for some of the costs that Medicare does not cover.

MEDICAID

Medicaid is a federal-state program that helps pay for health care for nonelderly people who are financially needy or who have a disability. Individual states determine who is eligible for Medicaid and which health services will be covered. Most people do not qualify for Medicaid until the majority of their money has been spent. It is important to realize, however, that some individuals whose incomes are not in the lowest category, but who have substantial medical expenses, do qualify for Medicaid. These individuals—who either have incomes higher than the AFDC (Aid for Families With Dependent Children) cut-off or have very high medical bills that drop their incomes below the level established for "categorically needy"—are termed "medically needy." Once an individual is covered by Medicaid, he or she is entitled to receive the following minimal services:

➤ Physician services

➤ Laboratory and X-ray services

➤ Outpatient hospital services

➤ Skilled nursing facilities (SNF) for persons over 21

➤ Family planning services

➤ Medical diagnosis and treatment for persons under 21

➤ Home health services for individuals

➤ Inpatient hospital service

In many states, Medicaid will also pay for some or all of the following:

➤ Dental care

➤ Medically necessary drugs

➤ Eyeglasses

➤ Prosthetic devices

➤ Physical, speech, and occupational therapy

➤ Private-duty nursing

➤ Alternative medical care, for example, chiropractors, acupuncturists

➤ Diagnostic, preventive, screening, and rehabilitative services

➤ Inpatient psychiatric care

Medicaid Waivers

Each state determines which services will be reimbursed by Medicaid. If you have any questions, contact your local social services agency.

Beginning in 1981, states have been able to obtain formal permission from the federal Medicaid agency (HCFA—Health Care Financing Administration) to set aside typical Medicaid restrictions. This permission allows for services to be provided in the home or community to certain individuals who would otherwise have to be institutionalized in order to be eligible for Medicaid.

Now in states with Medicaid waivers, children can stay at home when medically possible and, under certain conditions, not have their parents' income *deemed* (counted as belonging) to them. Also, under some waivers, some nonmedical services, such as respite care (discussed in Chapter 4), may now be covered by Medicaid.

The types of Medicaid waivers include the following:

Model Medicaid Waiver. Under this provision, states apply to the federal government for waivers before they can cover services traditionally covered by the Medicaid program in that state for persons who would have to be institutionalized. The requirement to consider income is waived to allow medically eligible persons to qualify for this program. Each state defines requirements for eligibility.

Home- and Community-Based Medical Waiver. Under this provision, states who apply to the federal government for waivers can cover services typically financed under Medicaid (as the Model Medicaid Waiver does) and go beyond to cover additional services in the community. These additional services are identified as "waivered services" in the community. Home- and community-based waivers are available for certain categories of individuals who otherwise would be institutionalized and who meet qualifications specified by the state for this waiver.

State Medicaid Plan Option. Another strategy states can use to help families become eligible for Medicaid is to amend the state plan. With this approach, states can provide, without obtaining special permission from the federal government, medical services to certain designated categories of children who would otherwise be institutionalized or hospitalized. Instead, a state plan, approved by the federal government, certifies categories of children who meet these qualifications.

FINAL WORD

As of the spring of 1996, vast changes have been made in the Welfare Reform Act. Consequently, each state is in the process of revising its legislation in accordance with the new federal guidelines. The ultimate effect will not be known for some time. It is clear, however, that in many cases, benefits will be diminished. Your individual situation should be explored with your local Department of Social Service and Social Security Administration.

Because of these changes, this may be a time to become proactive, or to renew your commitment to advocate for the needs of your family and your community.

— GLOSSARY —

ambulatory care facility—a facility that provides health care services (such as surgery) on an outpatient basis; an individual does not have to stay overnight.

ancillary services—laboratory tests, X-rays and all other hospital services other than room, board, and nursing service.

capitation—a set dollar limit that you or your employer pays to a health maintenance organization (HMO), regardless of how much you use (or don't use) the services offered by the health maintenance organization's providers.

case management—a system embraced by employers and insurance companies to ensure that individuals receive appropriate, reasonable health care services.

claim—a request by an individual (or his or her provider) to an individual's insurance company that the insurance company pay for services obtained from a health care professional.

COBRA—Consolidated Omnibus Budget Reconciliation Act of 1985 and its updates. Under this plan, businesses with more than twenty employees who offer health insurance must continue to make coverage of existing policies available at group rates for up to a period of eighteen months for employees who retire, quit, or are laid off. Those insured must pay the full cost of their insurance plus a 2 percent surcharge for administrative expenses.

co-insurance—money that an individual is required to pay for services, after a deductible has been paid. In some health care plans, co-insurance is called "copayment."

copayment—a predetermined (flat) fee that an individual pays for health care services, in addition to what the insurance covers.

deductible—the amount an individual must pay for health care expenses before insurance (or a self-insured company) covers the costs. Often, insurance plans are based on yearly deductible amounts.

denial of claim—refusal by an insurance company to honor a request by an individual (or his or her provider) to pay for health care services obtained from a health care professional.

employee assistance programs (EAPs)—Mental health counseling services that are sometimes offered by insurance companies or employers. Typically, individuals or employers do not have to pay directly for services provided through an employee assistance program.

exclusions—medical services that are not covered by an individual's insurance policy.

independent practice associations—IPAs are similar to HMOs, except that individuals receive care in a physician's own office, rather than in an HMO facility.

long-term care policy—an insurance policy that covers specified services for a specified period of time.

long-term disability—an injury or illness that keeps a person from working for a long time period.

LOS—Length of stay in a hospital or inpatient facility.

managed care—a medical delivery system that attempts to manage the quality and cost of medical services that individuals receive.

maximum dollar limit—the maximum amount of money that an insurance company (or self-insured company) will pay for claims within a specific time period.

open-ended HMOs—HMOs that allow enrolled individuals to use out-of-plan providers and still receive partial or full coverage and payment for the professional's services under a traditional indemnity plan.

out-of-plan—usually refers to physicians, hospitals, or other health care providers who are considered nonparticipants in an insurance plan (usually an HMO or PPO). Depending on an individual's health insurance plan, expenses of services provided by out-of-plan health professionals may not be covered, or may be covered only in part by an individual's insurance company.

out-of-pocket maximum—a predetermined, limited amount of money that an individual must pay out of his or her own savings, before an insurance company or (self-insured employer) will pay 100 percent for an individual's health care expenses.

outpatient—a patient who receives health care services (such as surgery) without staying overnight in a hospital or inpatient facility.

preadmission certification—also called precertification review, or preadmission review. Approval by a case manager or insurance company representative (usually a nurse) for a person to be admitted to a hospital or inpatient facility, granted prior to the admittance.

preadmission review—a review of an individual's health care status or condition, prior to admission to an inpatient health care facility, such as a hospital.

preadmission testing—medical tests that are completed for an individual prior to being admitted to a hospital or inpatient health care facility.

preexisting condition—a medical condition that is excluded from coverage by an insurance company, because the condition was believed to exist prior to the individual's obtaining a policy from the particular insurance company.

primary care provider (PCP)—a health care professional (usually a physician) responsible for monitoring an individual's overall health care needs.

provider —term used for health professionals who provide health care services.

reasonable and customary fee—the average fee charged by a particular type of health care practitioner within a geographic area. The term is often used by medical plans as the amount of money they will approve for a specific test or procedure.

risk—the chance of loss, the degree of probability of loss, or the amount of possible loss to the insuring company. For an individual, risk represents such probabilities as the likelihood of surgical complications, medications' side effects, exposure to infection, or the chance of suffering a medical problem because of a lifestyle or other choice.

second opinion—a medical opinion provided by a second medical expert, when one physician offers a diagnosis or recommends surgery to an individual.

second surgical opinion—an opinion provided by a second physician, when one physician recommends surgery to an individual.

short-term disability—an injury or illness that keeps a person from working for a short time. The definition of short-term disability (and the time period over which coverage extends) differs among insurance companies and employers.

triple-option—insurance plans that offer three options from which an individual may choose. Usually, the three options are: traditional indemnity, HMO, and PPO.

usual, customary, and reasonable (UCR) or covered expenses—an amount customarily charged for, or covered for, similar services and supplies that are medically necessary, recommended by a doctor, or required for treatment.

waiting period—a period of time when you are not covered by insurance for a particular problem.

workers' compensation —encompasses many different state and federal laws that provide financial benefits to workers and their families as compensation for work-related injuries, illnesses, diseases, and deaths. Time limits on filing claims differ by state. Employees who are injured on the job should notify their employer as soon as possible after an injury, and request and obtain appropriate treatment.

— REFERENCES —

Part A News, Part B News. United Communications Group, 11300 Rockville Pike, Rockville, MD 20852, (301)961-8700. Practical strategies for maximizing Medicare Part A and Part B.

Medicare Q & A. 5600 Fischers Lane, Rockville, MD 20857. Answers to commonly asked questions about Medicare.

— ORGANIZATIONS —

Social Security Library. U.S. Social Security Administration, P.O. Box 17330, Baltimore, MD 21235, (301)965-6113.

13

FINANCIAL CONCERNS

This chapter covers the following topics:

➤ Social Security Administration

➤ Supplemental Security Income (SSI)

➤ Criteria for determining SSI

➤ How to sign up for SSI benefits

➤ What to bring when signing up for SSI benefits

➤ Work incentives

➤ Social Security Disability Insurance (SSDI)

➤ Food stamps

ENTITLEMENT PROGRAMS

Many people with disabilities are eligible for benefits under one or more of several government programs. These programs are designed to protect the person with a disability by making sure that the person's financial resources are sufficient to provide the basic necessities of life—food, clothing, and health care.

To plan for the future of a child with disabilities, individuals must be aware of and use the many programs sponsored by the federal government and operated through a federal state partnership. These are called *entitlement programs*. Some of them are provided for large portions of the population in general—not just for persons with disabilities; other programs are specifically for people with disabilities. With a well-planned combination of services and, where possible, by supplementing these services with private assets, a parent can establish a relatively secure financial future for a son or daughter.

When it comes to parents' financing their children's future there are several paths that one can explore depending on the nature and severity of the child's disability and the personal assets of the family.

The following options should be explored and any one or a combination may be sufficient for a particular situation:

➤   using the family's own financial assets

➤   government assistance through a variety of programs

Since support from personal assets is self-explanatory, we will focus on the government programs that can provide financial support for individuals with disabilities.

SOCIAL SECURITY ADMINISTRATION

The Social Security Administration (SSA) directs two programs that can be of financial benefit to eligible individuals with disabilities throughout the transition process. These programs are:

➤   Supplemental Security Income (SSI) program

➤   Social Security Disability Insurance (SSDI) program

Because the Social Security Administration considers many variables before determining if a person is eligible for SSI or SSDI benefits, the discussion here is intended only as an overview to the benefits of these programs. Ultimately, an individual's eligibility can be determined only by contacting the Social Security Administration and filing an application.

SUPPLEMENTAL SECURITY INCOME (SSI)

The SSI program is targeted for individuals who are both (a) in financial need, and (b) blind or disabled. People who get SSI usually receive food stamps and Medicaid, too. The evaluation process to determine eligibility varies, depending upon whether the applicant is under the age of 18 or over. Recently, there have been many significant changes in how the SSA determines the SSI eligibility of individuals under the age of 18. These changes are expected to make it more difficult for children and youth with disabilities to qualify for SSI benefits. More information about these changes and the specific evaluation process the SSA now uses for individuals under the age of 18 is available by contacting the Social Security Administration directly. When a child reaches the age of 18, the Social Security Administration no longer considers the income and resources of parents in determining if the youth is eligible for benefits.

Under the SSI program, individuals over the age of 18 are eligible to receive monthly payments if they:

1.   have little or no income or resources such as savings accounts

2.   are considered medically disabled or blind

3.   do not work or earn less than a certain amount, defined by the Social Security Administration as substantial gainful activity (SGA).

Criteria for Determining SSI Benefits

To determine a person's financial need, the Social Security Administration considers the following:

➤ **The person's place of residence:** SSI payments may be reduced by different percentages, depending on the individual's residence. People who live in city or county rest homes, halfway houses, or other public institutions usually cannot get SSI checks, but there are some exceptions. A person living in a publicly operated community residence that serves no more than sixteen people may get SSI. Anyone living in a public institution mainly to attend approved educational or job training that will help him or her get a job may get SSI. Those living in a public emergency shelter for the homeless may be able to get SSI checks. If an individual lives in a public or private institution and Medicaid is paying more than half the cost of the care, he or she may get a small SSI check.

➤ **The parent's employment status:** An individual's SSI payments may be determined by parental income and employment status. This issue should be explored fully so that an individual with disability can receive the proper assistance.

➤ **Income and things owned by an individual with a disability:** Whether an individual can get SSI also depends on what he or she owns and how much income is coming in, such as wages, Social Security checks, and pensions. Income also includes such noncash items received as food, clothing, or shelter. If a person is married, the SSA will also look at the income of the spouse and the things the spouse owns. For someone under 18, SSA may look at the income of the parents and the things they own. For a sponsored alien, they may also look at the income of the sponsor and what he or she owns.

For specific information and criteria for any of the above factors contact your local Social Security Administration office.

Before an individual with a disability can get SSI, he or she must also meet other rules.

➤ One must live in the United States or Northern Mariana Islands.

➤ One must be a U.S. citizen or be in the United States legally.

➤ If one is eligible for Social Security or other benefits, then he or she must apply for them. (Eligible persons can get both SSI and Social Security checks if eligible for both.) If disabled, one must accept vocational rehabilitation services if they're offered.

How to Sign Up for SSI Benefits

Just visit the local Social Security office or call (800)772-1213 for an appointment with a Social Security representative who will help individuals sign up. SSI should be applied for right away; this benefit cannot start before the day one applies. Parents or guardians can apply for children under the age of 18 who are blind or disabled.

WHAT TO BRING WHEN SIGNING UP FOR SSI BENEFITS

Have the following things before applying for SSI benefits. Even if applicants don't have all of the things listed, however, sign up anyway. The people in the Social Security office are there to help applicants get whatever is needed.

➤ Social Security card or a record of Social Security number

➤   Birth certificate or other proof of age

➤   Information about residence, for example, a home with a mortgage or a lease and landlord's name

➤   Payroll slips, bank books, insurance policies, car registration, burial fund records, and other information about income and the things that are owned

➤   Medical information supporting the disability. When signing up for disability, the names, addresses, and telephone numbers of doctors, hospitals, and clinics are required. SSI checks can go directly into an individual's bank, so bring a checkbook or any other papers that show names and account numbers. Many people choose to have their checks sent to the bank because they find it safer and easier than getting their checks by mail.

WORK INCENTIVES

Most people with disabilities would rather work than try to live on disability benefits. There are a number of special rules for providing cash benefits and Medicare while they attempt to work. These rules are called *work incentives*. Be familiar with these disability work incentives so they can be used to the individual's advantage.

If an individual is receiving Social Security disability benefits, the following work incentives apply:

Trial Work Period: For nine months (not necessarily consecutive), people may earn as much as they can without affecting their benefits. (The nine months of work must fall within a five-year period before the trial work period can end.) A trial work month is any month in which they earn more than $200. After the trial work period ends, the work is evaluated to see if it is "substantial." If earnings do not average more than $500 a month, benefits will generally continue. If earnings do average more than $500 a month, benefits will continue for a three-month grace period before they stop.

Extended Period of Eligibility: For thirty-six months after a successful trial work period, an individual who is still disabled will be eligible to receive a monthly benefit without a new application for any month earnings drop below $500.

Deductions for Impairment-Related Expenses: Work expenses related to the disability will be discounted in figuring whether earnings constitute substantial work.

Medicare Continuation: Medicare coverage will continue for thirty-nine months beyond the trial work period. If Medicare coverage stops because of work, monthly premiums may be purchased.

Different rules apply to SSI recipients who work. For more information about Social Security and SSI work incentives, ask for a copy of the booklet, *Working While Disabled—How Social Security Can Help* (Publication No. 05-10095).

SOCIAL SECURITY DISABILITY INSURANCE (SSDI)

The SSDI program is a bit different, because it considers the employment status of the applicant's parents. "SSDI benefits are paid to persons who become disabled before the age of 22 if at least one of their parents had worked a certain amount of time under Social Security but is now disabled, retired, and/or deceased" (National Association of State Directors of Special Education 1990, p. 9). As with SSI, eligibility for SSDI generally makes an individual eligible for food stamps and Medicaid benefits as well.

Be aware that changes in legislation might result in a reduction of benefits. Recent legislation, however, has made major changes in both the SSI and SSDI programs to encourage people receiving these benefits to try to work and become independent. These changes are called work incentives, because they make it possible for individuals with disabilities to work without an immediate loss of benefits.

Whatever financial status a family has at the time a child turns 18, everyone involved should have a thorough knowledge of his or her financial entitlements.

FOOD STAMPS

The Food Stamp program provides financial assistance by enabling recipients to exchange the stamps for food. It is a major supplement for income if an individual with a disability meets the income requirements. This program is federally funded through the Department of Agriculture's Food and Nutrition Service (FNS). It is administered by state and local social service agencies. In most cases, if an individual is eligible for SSI, food stamps will be available too. For more information, contact your local department of social services.

A FINAL WORD

Dealing with the issue of entitlements is often frustrating, but it's important to persevere. For specific information about the benefits provided through SSDI and SSI contact your local Social Security Office (listed in the telephone directory under "Social Security Administration") and request a copy of the publications addressing SSI and SSDI. Single copies are free. You can also contact the SSA through its toll-free number: (800)234-5772 (voice) or (800)325-0778 (TDD); it is available 24 hours a day. Because of the volume of inquiries that SSA receives, it is best to call early in the morning or late in the afternoon. SSA also recommends calling later in the week.

— REFERENCES —

Booklets Available From the SSA

Social Security has many publications that contain information about other Social Security programs. Contact Social Security to get the most up-to-date, and free, copy of any of these publications. They include:

Understanding Social Security (Publication No. 05-10024). A comprehensive explanation of all the Social Security programs.

Retirement (Publication No. 05-10035). Explains Social Security retirement benefits.

Disability (Publication No. 05-10029). Explains Social Security disability benefits.

Medicare (Publication No. 10043). Explains Medicare hospital insurance and medical insurance.

Survivors (Publication No. 05-10084). Explains Social Security survivors' benefits.

Other References

Scarbourgh, D. *Helping You to Understand SSDI and SSI*. Accent Books and Products, P.O. Box 700, Bloomington, IL 61702, (800)787-8444.

A FINAL FEW WORDS

Remember, not every service is available and not every person can be helped 100 percent. Keep in mind that every year new programs begin and some old ones end, particularly at the state and local levels. Keep in touch with your contacts and stay as aware as you can, through reading and talking to knowledgeable people about what is happening in the area of services for individuals with disabilities. There are many excellent voluntary organizations as well as state, local, and federal offices that can help you. Numerous newsletters are produced by groups of and for individuals with disabilities. Using the Internet can connect people to much information and innumerable resources.

One of the major aspects of coping with a disability is educating oneself about both the disabling condition and what is available to enhance one's quality of life. Initially, the task of acquiring information falls to the families and the professionals they encounter. This information, however, must be passed on to the young person so that, as much as possible, he or she can achieve a satisfying independent life.

DISABILITIES NEWSLETTERS, MAGAZINES, AND JOURNALS

1. **ACLD Newsbriefs.** Learning Disabilities Association of America, 4156 Library Rd., Pittsburgh, PA 15234, (412)341-1515.

2. **Attention Magazine.** CHADD—Children With Attention Deficit Disorder, 499 NW 70th Avenue, Suite 109, Plantation, FL 33317, (800)233-4050 (voice mail to request information packet), (305)587-3700.

3. **ARC's Government Report.** Association for Retarded Citizens, 1522 K Street NW, Washington, DC 20005, (202)785-3388.

4. **Ability Magazine.** Jobs Information Business Service, 1682 Langley, Irvine, CA 92714, (714)854-8700; toll-free (800)453-JOBS.

5. **Case Manager.** Systemedic Corporation, 10809 Executive Center Drive, Suite 105, Little Rock, AR 72211, (501)227-5553.

6. **Choice Magazine.** 85 Channel Drive, Dept. 16, Port Washington, NY 11050, (516)883-8280. Free audio anthology available to visually impaired individuals, short stories, articles from over 100 sources.

7. **Closing the Gap** P.O. Box 68, Henderson, MN 56044, (612)248-3294. Assistive technology information.

8. **Dateline on Disability.** U.S. Department of Housing and Urban Development, Washington, DC 20410, (202)755-6422.

9. **Deaf American.** National Association of the Deaf, 814 Thayer Avenue, Silver Spring, MD 20910, (301)587-1788.

10. **Disabilities Resources Monthly.** Disabilities Resources, Inc., Four Glatter Lane, Centereach, NY 11720, (516)585-8290.

11. **Disabled Outdoors Magazine** HC 80, Box 395, Grand Marais, MN 55604, (218)387-9100.

12. **Exceptional Children.** Council for Exceptional Children, 1920 Association Drive, Reston, VA 22091, (703)620-3660; toll-free (800)232-7323.

13. **Exceptional Parent Magazine** 120 State Street, Hackensack, NJ 07601, (201)489-0871; toll-free (800)E-PARENT.

14. **First DIBS.** Disability Info. Brokerage System, P.O. Box 1285, Tucson, AZ 85702, (602)327-8277. Information resources for the consumer and others on disability topics.

15. **Hobby Newsnote.** P.O. Box 350073, Elmwood Park, IL 60635, (312)622-5996.

16. **ILRU Insights.** ILRU Research/Training Center for Independent Living, 2323 South Shepard, Suite 1000, Houston, TX 77019, (713)520-0232. National newsletter for independent living.

17. **JASH: The Journal of the Association for Persons With Severe Handicaps.** TASH, 11201 Greenwood Avenue, North Seattle, WA 98133, (206)361-8870.

18. **Journal of Speech and Hearing Disorders.** American Speech-Language-Hearing Association, 10801 Rockville Pike, Rockville, MD 20852, (301)897-5700.

19. **Journal of Visual Impairment and Blindness.** American Foundation for the Blind, 11 Penn Plaza, Suite 300, New York, NY 10001, (212)502-7600 (Voice); (212)502-7662 (TT); (800)232-5463.

20. **KALEIDOSCOPE: International Magazine of Literature, Fine Arts and Disability.** United Disability Services, 326 Locust Street, Akron, OH 44302, (216)762-9755.

21. **Life Lines.** Life Services for the Handicapped, Inc., 352 Park Avenue South, Suite 703, New York, NY 10010, (212)532-6740; toll-free (800)995-0066. Information about long-term care and planning for disabilities.

22. **Life Span.** National Council of Community Mental Health Centers, 12300 Twin Brook Parkway, Suite 320, Rockville, MD 20852, (301)984-6200. Information on tax tips, insurance, medical care, law and legislation.

23. **MDC Newsletter.** Materials Development Center, School of Education and Human Service, Menomonie, WI 54751. Information on employment and transition services.

24. **Mainstream Magazine.** 2973 Beech Street, San Diego, CA 92102, (619)234-3138. Reports on employment, education, new products and technology, etc.

25. **NARIC Quarterly.** National Rehabilitation Information Center, 8455 Colesville Rd., Suite 935, Silver Spring, MD 20910, (301)588-9284; toll-free (800)346-2742. Covers activities, projects, resources, and book reviews.

26. **NCD Bulletin.** National Council on Disabilities, 1331 F Street NW, Suite 1050, Washington, DC 20004, (202)272-2004. Covers latest issues on disabilities.

27. **National Council News.** National Council of Community Mental Health Centers, 12300 Twin Brook Parkway, Suite 320, Rockville, MD 20852, (301)984-6200. Information on legislation.

28. **National Networker.** National Network of Learning Disabled Adults, P.O. Box 32611, Phoenix, AZ 85064, (602)941-5112.

29. **Newsline.** Federation for Children With Special Needs, 95 Berkeley Street, Boston, MA 02116, (617)482-2195.

30. **NTID Focus.** National Technical Institute for the Deaf/RIT, P.O. Box 9887, 1 Lomb Memorial Drive, Rochester, NY 14623, (716)475-6400. Research on occupational aspects of deafness.

31. **On Our Own.** Vinfen Corporation—Gateway Crafts, 62 Harvard Street, Brookline, MA 02146, (617)734-1577. Journal by and for adults with developmental disabilities.

32. **PeopleNet.** P.O. Box 897, Levittown, NY 11756, (516)-579-4043. Information on relationships and sexuality, including personal ads.

33. **Pocket Guide to Federal Help for Individuals With Disabilities.** Consumer Information Center, Dept. 114A, Pueblo, CO 81009, (202)501-1794. Summary of benefits and services.

34. **Policy Updates.** Institute on Community Integration, 86 Pleasant Street, Wulling Hall, Minneapolis, MN 55455, (612)626-8200. Information on transition service issues.

35. **Recording for the Blind News.** 20 Roszel Rd., Princeton, NJ 08540, (609)452-0606; toll-free (800)221-4792.

36. **Volta Review.** Alexander Graham Bell Association, 3417 Volta Place NW, Washington, DC 20007, (202)337-5220. Professional journal.

NATIONAL ASSOCIATIONS AND ORGANIZATIONS

1. **Academic Therapy.** Contact Pro-Ed, 8700 Shoal Creek Boulevard, Austin, TX 78758-6897, (512)451-3246. Ask for the journal department.

2. **Accent on Information (AOI).** Gillum Road and High Drive, P.O. Box 700, Bloomington, IL 61702, (309)378-2961 (Voice). _Resource Useful to:_ Individuals with disabilities, families, professionals, service providers.

3. **Access Unlimited.** 3535 Briarpark Avenue, Suite 102, Houston, TX 77042, (713)781-7441; toll-free (800)848-0311. Information on personal computers and disability.

4. **Access/Abilities.** P.O. Box 458, Mill Valley, CA 94942, (415)388-3250 (Voice). _Resource Useful to:_ Families, individuals with disabilities, professionals, service providers.

5. **Accreditation Council on Services for People With Disabilities.** 8100 Professional Place, Suite 204, Landover, MD 20785, (301)459-3191 (Voice). _Resource Useful to:_ Agencies serving individuals with disabilities.

6. **Alexander Graham Bell Association for the Deaf.** 3417 Volta Place NW, Washington, DC 20007, (202)337-5220.

7. **Alliance for Technology Access.** 2175 East Francisco Boulevard, Suite L, San Rafael, CA 94901, (415)455-4575.

8. **Alliance of Genetic Support Groups.** 35 Wisconsin Circle, Suite 440, Chevy Chase, MD 20815, (800)336-4363; (301)652-5553.

9. **American Council of Rural Special Education (ACRES).** Department of Special Education, University of Utah, Milton Bennion Hall, Room 221, Salt Lake City, UT 84112, (801)581-8442.

10. **American Foundation for the Blind (AFB).** 11 Penn Plaza, Suite 300 New York, NY 10001, (212)502-7600 (Voice); (212)502-7662 (TT); (800)232-5463.

11. **American Occupational Therapy Association (AOTA).** P.O. Box 31220, 4720 Montgomery Lane, Bethesda, MD 20824-1220, (301)652-2682; (800)377-8555 (TT).

12. **American Physical Therapy Association (APTA).** 1111 North Fairfax Street, Alexandria, VA 22314, (703)684-2782; (800)999 2782.

13. **American Self-Help Clearinghouse.** St. Clare's Community Health Center, Denville, NJ 07834, (800)367-6274. A clearinghouse that makes referrals to self-help groups throughout the nation.

14. **American Speech-Language-Hearing Association (ASHA).** 10801 Rockville Pike, Rockville, MD 20852, (301)897-5700 (Voice/TT); (800)638-8255.

15. **American Therapeutic Recreation Association.** P.O. Box 15215 Hattiesburg, MS 39404-5215 (800)553-0304

16. **ARC (formerly the Association for Retarded Citizens).** National Headquarters, 500 E. Border Street, Arlington, TX 76010, (817)261-6003. *Resources Useful for:* Parents, professionals.

17. **ARCH National Resource Center.** Crisis Nurseries and Respite Care Services, Chapel Hill Training—Outreach Project, 800 Eastowne Drive, Suite 105, Chapel Hill, NC 27514 (800)473-1727 (Voice toll-free); (919)490-5577 (Voice). *Resource Useful to:* Crisis nurseries and respite care providers, parents, advocates, caregivers.

18. **ASHA.** Contact the American Speech-Language-Hearing Association, 10801 Rockville Pike, Rockville, MD 20852, (301)897-5700, extension 218.

19. **Association for the Care of Children's Health (ACCH).** 7910 Woodmont Avenue, Suite 300, Bethesda, MD 20814-3015, (301)654-6549.

20. **Association for Persons With Severe Handicaps.** 29 W. Susquehanna Avenue, Suite 210, Baltimore, MD 21204, (410)828-8274. *Resource Useful to:* Parents, advocates, educators, other professionals.

21. **Association for the Advancement of Rehabilitation Technology.** 1700 North Moore St., Suite 1540, Arlington, VA 22209-1903, (703)524-6686 (Voice); (703)524-6639 (TT).

22. **Association for the Care of Children's Health.** 7910 Woodmont Avenue, Suite 300, Bethesda, MD 20814, (301)654-6549 (Voice). *Resource Useful to:* Health professionals, parents, educators.

23. **Autism Society of America (formerly NSAC).** 7910 Woodmont Avenue, Suite 650, Bethesda, MD 20814, (301)657-0881; (800)3-AUTISM. Fact sheet available in Spanish.

24. **Beach Center on Families and Disability.** University of Kansas, 3111 Haworth Hall, Lawrence, KS 66045, (913)864-7600 (Voice/TT). *Resource Useful to:* Families, individuals with disabilities, service providers, professionals.

25. **Brain Injury Association.** (formerly the National Head Injury Foundation), 1776 Massachusetts Avenue NW, Suite 100, Washington, DC 20036, (202)296-6443.

26. **CAPP National Parent Resource Center.** Federation for Children With Special Needs, 95 Berkeley Street, Suite 104, Boston, MA 02116, (617)482-2915 (Voice/TT); (800)331-0688 (toll-free in MA). *Resource Useful to:* Parents, health agencies and departments, other agencies.

27. **Center for Children With Chronic Illness and Disability.** Division of General Pediatrics and Adolescent Health, University of Minnesota, 420 Delaware Street, Minneapolis, MN 55455, (612)626-4032 (Voice); (612)624-3939 (TT). *Resource Useful to:* Families; health, education, social services and advocates.

28. **Center for Human Disabilities.** George Mason University, Fairfax, VA 22030, (703)993-3670 (Voice/TT). *Resource Useful to:* Special educators, related services providers, special education administrators, parents, policymakers.

29. **Child and Adolescent Service System Program Technical Assistance Center.** Georgetown University, 2233 Wisconsin Avenue NW, Suite 215, Washington, DC 20007, (202)338-1831 (Voice). *Resource Useful to:* Mental health service providers, families.

30. **Children and Adults With Attention Deficit Disorders (CHADD).** 499 NW 70th Avenue, Suite 109, Plantation, FL 33317.

31. **Clearinghouse on Disability Information.** Office of Special Education and Rehabilitative Services (OSERS), Room 3132, Switzer Building, 330 C Street SW, Washington, DC 20202-2524, (202)205-8241 (Voice/TT). *Resource Useful to:* Individuals with disabilities, families, agencies, information providers, and others.

32. **Coalition on Sexuality and Disability, Inc.** 122 East 23rd Street, New York, NY 10010, (212)-242-3900 TTY/TTD; (212)677 6474. *Resources Useful to:* Educators, parents, advocates.

33. **Complete Directory for People With Disabilities.** 1995 Grey House Publishing, Pocket Knife Square, Lakeville, CT 06039, (800)562-2139; (203)435-0868; Fax (203)435-0867.

34. **Council for Exceptional Children (CEC).** 1920 Association Drive, Reston, VA 22091-1589, (703)620-3660 (Voice/TT). *Resource Useful to:* Teachers, administrators, students, parents, related services personnel, and others working with individuals with disabilities and those who are gifted.

35. **Courage Center.** 3915 Golden Valley Road, Golden Valley, MN 55422, (612)588-0811 (Voice); (612)520-0520 (Voice); (612)520-0401 (TT). *Resource Useful to:* Persons with disabilities, parents.

36. **Developmental Disability Councils.** 200 Independence Avenue SW, Washington, DC 20201, (202)245-2890. Councils in each state provide training and technical assistance to local and state agencies.

37. **DIRECT LINK for the Disabled, Inc.** P.O. Box 1036, Solvang, CA 93464, (805)688-1603 (Voice/TT). *Resource Useful to:* Families, individuals with disabilities, service providers.

38. **Disability Statistics Program Information Services Institute for Health and Aging.** University of California, San Francisco, N 631Y, Box 0612, San Francisco, CA 94143-0612, (415)788-8916 (Voice/TT). *Resource Useful to:* Families, students, researchers.

39. **Disability Statistics Rehabilitation Research and Training Center (RRTC).** Institute for Health and Aging, UCSF, 3333 California St., Rm. 340, San Francisco, CA 94118, (415)502-5210; (415)502-5208 (Fax).

40. **Epilepsy Foundation of America (EFA).** 4351 Garden City Drive, 5th Floor, Landover, MD 20785, (301)459-3700; (800)332-1000. Publications available in Spanish; Spanish speaker on staff.

41. **ERIC Clearinghouse on Disabilities and Gifted Education.** Council for Exceptional Children (CEC), 1920 Association Drive, Reston, VA 22091, (703)264-9474 (Voice); (703)620-3660 (TT). *Resource Useful to:* Teachers, administrators, policymakers, parents, researchers, students.

42. **Family Resource Center on Disabilities.** 20 East Jackson Boulevard, Room 900, Chicago, IL 60604, (800)952-4199 (Voice toll-free); (312)939-3513 (Voice, local); (312)939-3519 (TT). *Resource Useful to:* Parents, professionals.

43. **Federation for Children With Special Needs.** 95 Berkeley Street, Boston, MA 02116, (617)482-2915 (Voice/TT); (800)331-0688 (toll-free in MA). *Resource Useful to:* Parents, professionals.

44. **Federation of Families for Children's Mental Health.** 1021 Prince Street, Alexandria, VA 22314-2971, (703)684-7710 (Voice). *Resource Useful to:* Parents, professionals.

45. **Focal Point.** Contact Portland State University, Research and Training Center on Family Support and Children's Mental Health, Regional Research Institute for Human Services, P.O. Box 751, Portland, OR 97207-0751, (503)725-4040.

46. **Gallaudet University.** 800 Florida Avenue NE, Washington, DC 20002, (800)451-1073.

47. **Goodwill Industries International.** 9200 Wisconsin Avenue, Bethesda, MD 20814, (301)530-6500. Provides occupational opportunities.

48. **Handicapper Educational Services.** Wayne State University, 583 Student Center Building, Detroit, MI 48202, (313)577-1851. Advocacy services for students with disabilities.

49. **HEATH Resource Center.** 1 Dupont Circle, Suite 800, Washington, DC 20036, (800)544-3284. National Clearinghouse for information on postsecondary education for people with disabilities.

50. **Helen Keller National Center for Deaf and Blind Youth Adults.** 111 Middle Neck Rd., Sands Point, NY 90057, (213)483-4431.

51. **Independent Living Research Utilization Project (ILRU).** The Institute for Rehabilitation and Research, 2323 South Sheppard, Suite 1000, Houston, TX 77019, (713)520-0232; (713)520-5136 (TT).

52. **International Council on Disability.** 25 East 21st Street, New York, NY 10010, (212)420-1500.

53. **International Resource Center for Down Syndrome.** Keith Building 1621 Euclid Avenue, Suite 514, Cleveland, OH 44115, (216)621-5858; (800)899-3039 (in OH only).

54. **International Rett Syndrome Association.** 9121 Piscataway Road, Suite 2B, Clinton, MD 20735, (301)856-3334. Publication "What Is Rhett Syndrome?" available in Spanish.

55. **Journal of Learning Disabilities.** Contact Pro-Ed, 8700 Shoal Creek Boulevard, Austin, TX 78758-6897, (512)451-3246. Ask for the journal department.

56. **Learning Disability Association of America (LDA) (formerly ACLD).** 4156 Library Road, Pittsburgh, PA 15234, (412)341-1515; (412)341-8077. Publications available in Spanish.

57. **Lexington Center, Inc.** 30th Avenue & 75th Street, Jackson Heights, NY 11370, (718)899-8800. Offers a comprehensive range of services and materials for the deaf.

58. **Lighthouse, Inc.** 111 East 59th Street, New York, NY 10022, (800)334-5497. Vision rehabilitation organization.

59. **March of Dimes Birth Defects Foundation.** 1275 Mamaroneck Avenue, White Plains, NY 10605, (914) 428-7100. Publications available in Spanish; Spanish speaker on staff.

60. **Muscular Dystrophy Association (MDA).** 3300 East Sunrise Drive, Tucson, AZ 85718, (602)529-2000. Publications available in Spanish; Spanish speaker on staff.

61. **National Alliance for the Mentally Ill (NAMI).** 200 N. Glebe Road, Suite 1015, Arlington, VA 22203-3754, (703)524-7600; (800)950-NAMI.

62. **National Association of Private Schools for Exceptional Children (NAPSEC).** 1522 K Street NW, Suite 1032, Washington, DC 20005, (202)408-3338.

63. **National Association of the Deaf.** 814 Thayer Avenue, Silver Spring, MD 20910, (301)587-1788.

64. **National Center for Education in Maternal and Child Health.** 2000 15th Street N., Ste. 701, Arlington, VA 22201, (703)524-7802. Information service on children with special health needs.

65. **National Center for Learning Disabilities (NCLD).** 381 Park Avenue South, Suite 1420, New York, NY 10016, (212)545-7510.

66. **National Center for Youth With Disabilities.** University of Minnesota, Box 721, 420 Delaware Street SE, Minneapolis, MN 55455, (800)333-6293. Information, policy, and resource center.

67. **National Clearinghouse on Family Support and Children's Mental Health.** Portland State University, P.O. Box 751, Portland, OR 97207-0751, (800)628-1696 (toll-free); (503)725-4040 (local); (503)725-4165 (TT). *Resource Useful to:* Professionals, families whose children have behavioral or emotional disorders.

68. **National Coalition for Parent Involvement in Education (NCPIE).** 1201 16th Street NW, Room 810, Washington, DC 20036, (800)695-0285 (Voice/TT). *Resource Useful to:* Educational organizations, professionals.

69. **National Coalition of Title I Chapter I Parents.** Edmonds School Building, 9th & D Street NE, Washington, DC 20002, (202)547-9286 (Voice). *Resource Useful to:* Parents.

70. **National Council on Disability (NCD).** 1331 F Street NW, Washington, DC 20004-1107, (202)267-3846 (Voice); (202)267-3232 (TT). *Resource Useful to:* Policymakers, individuals with disabilities.

71. **National Down Syndrome Congress.** 1605 Chantilly Drive, Suite 250, Atlanta, GA 30324, (404) 633-1555; (800)232-6372 (toll-free). Pamphlet available in Spanish; Spanish speaker on staff.

72. **National Down Syndrome Society.** 666 Broadway, New York, NY 10012, (212)460-9330; (800) 221-4602. Publications available in Spanish; Spanish speaker on staff.

73. **National Easter Seal Society.** 230 West Monroe Street, Chicago, IL 60603, (312)726-6200 (Voice); (312)726-4258 (TT). *Resource Useful to:* Organizations, Easter Seal affiliates, individuals.

74. **National Federation for the Blind.** 1800 Johnson Street, Baltimore, MD 21230, (800)638-7518.

75. **National Fragile X Foundation.** 1441 York Street, Suite 303, Denver, CO 80206, (800)688-8765; (303)333-6155.

76. **National Information Center for Children and Youth With Disabilities (NICHCY).** P.O. Box 1492, Washington, DC 20013, (800)695-0285 (Voice/TT). *Resource Useful to:* Parents, educators, service providers, individuals with disabilities.

77. **National Information Center on Deafness.** Gallaudet University Bookstore, 800 Florida Avenue NE, Washington, DC 20002, (800)451-1073.

78. **National Information Clearinghouse (NIC) for Infants With Disabilities and Life-Threatening Conditions.** Center for Developmental Disabilities, University of South Carolina, Columbia, SC 29208, (800)922-9234, ext. 201 (Voice/TT). *Resource Useful to:* Parents, educators, service providers, individuals with disabilities.

79. **National Institute on Disability and Rehabilitation Research (NIDRR).** 330 C Street SW, Washington, DC 20202, (202)205-9151 (Voice); (202)205-9136 (TT). *Resource Useful to:* Professionals, administrators, rehabilitation specialists.

80. **National Library Services for the Blind & Physically Handicapped.** The Library of Congress, Washington, DC 20542, (202)707-5100; (202)707-0744 (TTY); (800)424-8567; (800)424-9100 (TTY, English); (800)345-8901 (TTY, Spanish).

81. **National Organization on Disability.** 910 Sixteenth Street NW, Washington, DC 20006, (202)293-5960. Helps promote full participation for individuals with disabilities.

82. **National Organization on Rare Disorders (NORD).** 100 Rt. 37, P.O. Box 8923, New Fairfield, CT 06812-1783, (800)999-6673 (Voice toll-free); (203)746-6518 (Voice, local); (203)746-6927 (TT). *Resource Useful to:* Parents, professionals.

83. **National Parent to Parent.** P.O. Box 907, Ridge, GA 30513, (800)651-1151. nnppsis@aol.com.

84. **National Spinal Cord Injury Association.** 545 Concord Avenue, Cambridge, MA 02138, (617)441-8500; (800)962-9629. Publications available in Spanish; Spanish speaker on staff.

85. **National Technical Institute for the Deaf.** LBJ Building, 52 Lomb Memorial Drive, Rochester, NY 14623, (716)475-6400.

86. **National Transition Network.** Institute on Community Integration (UAP), University of Minnesota, Pettee Hall, 150 Pillsbury Drive. SE, Minneapolis, MN 55455, (612)626-8200. *Resources Useful to:* parents, professionals.

87. **New York State Journal of Medicine.** Contact the Medical Society of the State of New York, 420 Lakeville Road, Box 5404, Lake Success, NY 11042-1160, (516)488-6100.

88. **Office of Special Populations.** National Center for Research in Vocational Education, University of Illinois, Suite 345, Education Building, 1310 South 6th Street, Champaign, IL 61820, (217)333-0807 (Voice). *Resource Useful to:* Vocational and special educators; administrators.

89. **Orton Dyslexia Society.** Chester Building # 382, 8600 LaSalle Road, Baltimore, MD 21286, (410)296-0232; toll-free (800)222-3123.

90. **Osteogenesis Imperfecta Foundation.** 5005 W. Laurel Street, Suite 210, Tampa, FL 33607, (800)981-BONE.

91. **Parent Care.** 9041 Colgate Street, Indianapolis, IN 46268-1210, (317)872-9913 (Voice). *Resource Useful to:* Parents, perinatal professionals, advocates.

92. **Parent Training and Information (PTI) Centers.** *Resource Useful to:* Parents and families. To find out about the PTI for your state, you can either call NICHCY at (800)695-0285, or contact the Technical Assistance for Parent Programs (TAPP) at (617)482-2915. TAPP is described below.

93. **Parents Advocacy Coalition for Educational Rights (PACER).** PACER Center, Inc., 4826 Chicago Avenue South, Minneapolis, MN 55417, (612)827-2966 (Voice/TDD). *Resources Useful to:* Parents and advocates.

94. **Parents Helping Parents.** The Parent-Directed Family Resource Center for Children With Special Needs, 535 Race Street, Suite 140, San Jose, CA 95126, (408)288-5010 (Voice). *Resource Useful to:* Parents, professionals, self-help support groups serving children with special needs.

95. **President's Committee's Job Accommodation Network (JAN).** West Virginia University, 918 Chestnut Ridge Road, Suite 1, P.O. Box 6080, Morgantown, WV 26506-6080, (800)526-7234 (Voice/TT, toll-free in U.S.); (800)526-2262 (Voice/TT, toll-free in Canada). Publications available in Spanish.

96. **Recording for the Blind and Dyslexic.** The Anne T. Macdonald Center, 20 Roszel Road Princeton, NJ 08540, (800)221-4792; (609)452-0606 and 5022 Hollywood Blvd. Los Angeles, CA 90027, (213)644-5525. Publications available in Spanish; Spanish speaker on staff.

97. **Sexuality and Disability.** Contact J. S. Canner & Company, Inc., 10 Charles Street, Needham Heights, MA 02194, (617)449-9103.

98. **Sibling Information Network.** A. J. Pappanikou Center, University of Connecticut, 249 Glenbrook Road, U64, Storrs, CT 06269-2064, (860)486-5035. Spanish speaker on staff.

99. **Sick Kids (need) Involved People (SKIP).** 545 Madison Avenue, 13th Floor, New York, NY 10022. (212)421-9160; (212)421-9161. Spanish speaker on staff.

100. **SIECUS Report.** Contact SIECUS, 130 West 42nd Street, Suite 2500, New York, NY 10036, (212)819-9770.

101. **Special Olympics.** 1325 G Street NW, Suite 500, Washington, DC 20005, (202)628-3630. Publications available in Spanish and French; Spanish-French speaker on staff.

102. **Special Parent/Special Child.** Contact Lindell Press, Inc., P.O. Box 462, South Salem, NY 10590.

103. **Spina Bifida Association of America.** 4590 MacArthur Boulevard NW, Suite 250, Washington, DC 20007, (202)944-3285; (800)621-3141. Publications available in Spanish.

104. **Teaching Exceptional Children.** Contact Council for Exceptional Children, 1920 Association Drive, Reston, VA 22091-1589, (703)620-3660. Ask for Publications Department.

105. **Technical Assistance for Parent Programs (TAPP).** Federation for Children With Special Needs, 95 Berkeley Street, Suite 104, Boston, MA 02116, (617)482-2915 (Voice/TT); *Resource Useful to:* Parent Training and Information (PTI) Centers, parent groups, parents.

106. **Trace Research & Development Center.** S-151 Waisman Center, 1500 Highland Avenue, University of Wisconsin-Madison, Madison, WI 53705-2280, (608)262-6966; (608)263-5408 (TT).

107. **United Cerebral Palsy Association, Inc.** 1660 L Street NW, Suite 700, Washington, DC 20036, (202)842-1266; (800)872-5827. Publications available in Spanish.

108. **Very Special Arts.** 1331 F Street NW, Ste. 800, Washington, DC 20004, (800)933-8721. Provides leadership and support for individuals with disabilities to develop artistic expression.

109. **Young Adults Institute.** 460 West 34th Street, New York, NY 10001, (212)563-7474.

DISABILITY INTERNET SITES

ARC (formerly the Association for Retarded Citizens). National Headquarters, 500 E. Border Street, Arlington, TX 76010, (817)261-6003.
URL: http://www.thearc.org/welcome.html

BEACH Center (excellent resource for parents).
URL: http://www.lsi. ukans.edu/beach/beachhp.htm

Children and Adults With Attention Deficit Disorders (CHADD). 499 NW 70th Avenue, Suite 109, Plantation, FL 33317.
URL: http://www. chadd.org/

Council for Exceptional Children (CEC). 1920 Association Drive, Reston, VA 22091-1589, (703)620-3660 (Voice/TT).
URL: http://www.cec.sped.org/home.htm

ERIC Clearinghouse on Disabilities & Gifted Education. Council for Exceptional Children (CEC), 1920 Association Drive, Reston, VA 22091-1589, (703)487-9432; (800)328-0272; (703)264-9449 (TTY).
URL: http://www.cec.sped.org/er-menu.htm

HEATH Resource Center (National Clearinghouse on Postsecondary Education for Individuals With Disabilities). One Dupont Circle NW, Suite 800, Washington, DC. 20036-1193, (202)939-9320; (800)544-3284 (Voice/TTY).
Gopher: //hawking u. washington.edu/11/disability realted/health

National Alliance for the Mentally Ill (NAMI) (a significant organization for families). 200 N. Glebe Rd., Suite 1015, Arlington, VA 22203, (800)950-0264.
URL: http://www.nami.org/no frames.htm

National Center for Learning Disabilities (NCLD). 381 Park Avenue South, Suite 1420, New York, NY 10016, (212)545-7510.
URL: http://www.ncld.org

National Information Center for Children and Youth With Disabilities (NICHCY). P.O. Box 1492, Washington, DC 20013, (800)695-0285 (Voice/TT).
URL: http://www. aed.org/nichcy/pag1.html

National Rehabilitation Information Center (NARIC). 8455 Colesville Road, Suite 935, Silver Spring, MD 20910-3319, (301)588-9284; (800)227-0216 (Voice/TT). Spanish speaker on staff.
URL: http://www.naric.com/naric

National Transition Alliance.
URL: http/www. aed. org/transition/alliance/nta.html

Parents Advocacy Coalition for Educational Rights (PACER). PACER Center, Inc., 4826 Chicago Avenue South, Minneapolis, MN 55417, (612)827-2966 Voice and TDD.
URL: http://www.

Special Education Resources on the Internet (SERI). One of the most extensive resources of interest to those involved in the field of special education.
URL: http/www. hood.edu/serihome.htm

Appendix D

GENERAL INFORMATION ABOUT AGENCIES

OFFICES OF STATE COORDINATOR OF VOCATIONAL EDUCATION FOR STUDENTS WITH DISABILITIES

States receiving federal funds used for vocational education must ensure that funding is used in programs that include students with disabilities. This office can tell you how your state funds are being used and provide you with information on current programs.

PROGRAMS FOR CHILDREN WITH SPECIAL HEALTH CARE NEEDS

The U.S. Department of Health and Human Services, Maternal and Child Health Bureau, provides grants to states for direct medical and related services to children with handicapping conditions. Although services will vary from state to state, additional federal programs may be funded for training, research, special projects, genetic disease testing, and counseling services. For additional information about current grants and programs in your state, contact the National Center for Education in Maternal and Child Health, 2000 N. 15th Street, Suite 701, Arlington, VA 22201-2617. Telephone: (703)524-7802.

STATE DEVELOPMENTAL DISABILITIES COUNCILS

Assisted by the U.S. Department of Health and Human Services, Administration on Developmental Disabilities, state councils plan and advocate for improvement in services for people with developmental disabilities. In addition, funding is made available for time-limited demonstration and stimulatory grant projects.

STATE EDUCATION DEPARTMENTS

The State Department staff can answer questions about special education and related services in your state. Many states have special manuals explaining the steps to take. Check to see if one is available. State Department officials are responsible for special education and related services programs in their state for preschool, elementary, and secondary age children.

STATE MENTAL HEALTH AGENCIES

The functions of state mental health agencies vary from state to state. The general purposes of these offices are to plan, administer, and develop standards for state and local mental health programs such as state hospitals and community health centers. They can provide information to the consumer about mental illness and a resource list of where you can go for help.

211

STATE MENTAL RETARDATION/DEVELOPMENTAL DISABILITIES AGENCIES

The functions of state mental retardation/developmental disabilities agencies vary from state to state. The general purpose of this office is to plan, administer, and develop standards for state/local mental retardation/developmental disabilities programs provided in state-operated facilities and community-based programs. This office provides information about available services to families, consumers, educators, and other professionals.

STATE PROTECTION AND ADVOCACY AGENCY AND CLIENT ASSISTANCE PROGRAM

Protection and advocacy systems are responsible for pursuing legal, administrative, and other remedies to protect the rights of people who have developmental disabilities or mental illness, regardless of their age. Protection and advocacy agencies may provide information about health, residential, and social services in your area. Legal assistance is also available. The Client Assistance Program provides assistance to individuals seeking and receiving vocational rehabilitation services. These services, provided under the Rehabilitation Act of 1973, include assisting in the pursuit of legal, administrative, and other appropriate remedies to ensure the protection of the rights of individuals with developmental disabilities.

STATE VOCATIONAL REHABILITATION AGENCIES

The state vocational rehabilitation agency provides medical, therapeutic, counseling, education, training, and other services needed to prepare people with disabilities for work. This state agency will provide you with the address of the nearest rehabilitation office where you can discuss issues of eligibility and services with a counselor. The state vocational rehabilitation agency can also refer you to an independent living program in your state. Independent living programs provide services that enable adults with disabilities to live productively as members of their communities. The services might include, but are not limited to, information and referral, peer counseling, workshops, attendant care, and technical assistance.

UNIVERSITY-AFFILIATED PROGRAMS (UAPs)

A national network of programs affiliated with universities and teaching hospitals, UAPs provide interdisciplinary training for professionals and paraprofessionals and offer programs and services for children with disabilities and their families. Individual UAPs have staff with expertise in a variety of areas and can provide information, technical assistance, and inservice training to agencies, service providers, parent groups, and others. You can obtain information about University-Affiliated Programs, as well as a listing of all UAPs, by contacting American Association of University Affiliated Programs for Persons With Developmental Disabilities (AAUAP), 8630 Fenton Street, Suite 410, Silver Spring, MD 20910, (301)588-8252.

SELECTED GOVERNMENT AGENCIES

1. **Equal Opportunity Employment Commission.** 1801 L Street NW, Washington, DC 20507, (800)669-4000.

2. **Health Care Financing Administration.** 200 Independence Avenue NW, Washington, DC 20410, (202)245-6726.

3. **Independent Living Office.** 451 7th Street SW, Washington, DC 20410, (202)755-5866.

4. **National Council on Disability.** 1331 F Street NW, Suite 1050, Washington, DC 20004, (202)272-2004.

5. **Office of Special Education Programs, Department of Education.** 330 C Street SW, Room 3086, Washington, DC 20202, (202)732-1007.

6. **President's Committee on Mental Retardation.** 330 Independence Avenue SW, Washington, DC 20201, (202)619-0634.

7. **Protection and Advocacy Program for the Mentally Ill.** U.S. Department of Health and Human Services, 5600 Fishers Lane, Room 11-C-22, Rockville, MD 20852, (301)443-3667.

8. **Protection and Advocacy for Persons With Developmental Disabilities.** U.S. Department of Health and Human Services, 5600 Fishers Lane, Room 11-C-22, Rockville, MD 20852, (301)443-3667.

9. **Social Security Administration.** 6401 Security Blvd., Baltimore, MD 21202, (800)772-1213.

10. **U.S. Department of Transportation.** 400 7th Street SW, Washington, DC 20590, (202)366-9305.

SCHOLARSHIP AND FINANCIAL AID RESOURCES

Scholarships specifically designated for students with disabilities are extremely limited. Listed below are organizations that offer the few disability specific scholarships.

Alexander Graham Bell Association of the Deaf. 3417 Volta Place NW, Washington, DC 20007, (202)337-5220 (Voice/TT).

American Council of the Blind. 1155 15th Street NW, Suite 720, Washington, DC 20005, (800)424-8666 (3:00-5:30 P.M.); (202)467-5081.

American Foundation for the Blind. 15 West 16th Street, New York, NY 10011, (800)232-5463; (212)620-2000.

Association for Education and Rehabilitation of the Blind and Visually Impaired. 206 North Washington Street, Suite 320, Alexandria, VA 22314, (703)548-1884.

Bridge Endowment Fund. Scholarship Office, National FFA (Future Farmers of America) Center, P.O. Box 15160, Alexandria, VA 22309-0160, (703)360-3600.

Blinded Veterans Association. 477 H St. NW, Washington, DC 20001-2694, (202)371-8880. For children and spouses of blinded veterans.

Central Intelligence Agency (CIA). Office of Student Programs (Internships), P.O. Box 1925, Department T, Room 220, Washington, DC 20013, (703)281-8365.

Christian Record Braille Foundation. 4444 South 52nd Street, Lincoln, NE 68506, (402)488-0981.

Council of Citizens With Low Vision (CCLV). 5707 Brockton Drive, No. 302, Indianapolis, IN 46220, (317)254-0185; (800)733-2258.

Electronic Industries Foundation (EIF). 919 18th Street NW, Suite 900, Washington, DC 20006, (202)955-5814; (TDD 955-5836). Contact Marcie Vorac (technical or scientific field).

Foundation for Exceptional Children. 1920 Association Drive, Reston, VA 22091, (703)620-1054.

Foundation for Science and Disability, Inc. Rebecca F. Smith, 115 S. Brainard Avenue, La Grange, IL 60525. For science students with a disability studying for a master's degree.

The Geoffrey Foundation. P.O. Box 1112, Ocean Avenue, Kennebunkport, ME 04046, (207)967-5798. Offered to hearing-impaired auditory-verbal children and students.

Graduate Fellowship Fund. Gallaudet University Alumni Association, Alumni Office, Gallaudet University, 800 Florida Avenue NE, Washington, DC 20002, (202)651-5060 (Voice/TT). Limited to Ph.D. students who are hearing impaired.

Immune Deficiency Foundation. 3566 Ellicott Mills Drive, Unit B2, Ellicott City, MD 21043. Limited to those with primary genetic immune deficiency.

Jewish Braille Institute of America. 110 E. 30th Street, New York, NY 10016. Offered to students who wish to become rabbis, cantors, or Jewish educators.

La Sertoma International. 1912 E. Meyer Boulevard, Kansas City, MO 64312, (816)333-3116. Limited to graduate students preparing to assist people who are blind.

Lighthouse, Inc. 800 2nd Avenue, New York, NY 10017. Legally blind students.

National Association of the Deaf. Stokoe Scholarship (supports research related to sign language or deafness). 814 Thayer Avenue, Silver Spring, MD 20910, (301)587-1788 (Voice), (301)587-1789 (TT).

National Captioning Institute, Inc. Dr. Malcolm J. Norwood, Memorial Award Panel, 5203 Leesburg Pike, Suite 1500, Falls Church, VA 22041, (703)998-2400 (Voice/TT). Limited to students studying for careers in communication or media technology.

National Federation of the Blind. 1800 Johnson Street, Baltimore, MD 21230, (410)659-9314.

National Federation of Music Clubs. Music for the Blind Department, 55 Janssen Place, Kansas City, MO 64109.

National Hemophilia Foundation. 110 Greene Street, New York, NY 10012, (800)42-HANDI.

National 4-H Council. 7100 Connecticut Avenue, Chevy Chase, MD 20815, (301)961-2800.

Opportunities for the Blind. P.O. Box 510, Leonardtown, MD 20650.

The President's Committee on Employment of People With Disabilities. 1331 F Street NW, Washington, DC 20004, (202)376-6200.

Recording for the Blind. 20 Rozelle Road, Princeton, NJ 08540, (609)452-0606.

Spina Bifida Association of America. 4590 MacArthur Boulevard NW, Suite 250, Washington, DC 20007, (800)621-3141; (202)944-3285.

Trapshooting Hall of Fame College Scholarship Fund Chairshooters. 161 Fort Washington Avenue, New York, NY 10032, (212)305-5559. Contact: Hugo A. Keim, M.D.

Venture Clubs Student Aid Award and Venture Clubs Handicapped Student Scholarship Fund. 1616 Walnut Street, Suite 700, Philadelphia, PA 19103, (215)732-0512.

Very Special Arts Education Office. John F. Kennedy Center for the Performing Arts, Washington, DC 20566. Limited to students age 10-21 studying selected musical instruments.

The International Kiwanis Club recommends checking with local Kiwanis organizations to see if they offer scholarships. To find the number of the local chapter, call (317)875-8755.

The Elks Grand Lodge in Winton, NC, may be contacted for scholarships at (919)358-7661.

The Rotary Club offers scholarships and may be contacted at (202)638-3555 for more information. Scholarships must be applied for two years in advance.

PUBLISHERS—BOOKS AND VIDEOS ON ISSUES DEALING WITH DISABILITIES

The publishers listed below are only some of the many that provide information about issues relating to individuals with disabilities, for example, social skills, sexuality, and sexuality education.

1.   **Active Parenting, Inc.** 810 Franklin Court, Suite B, Marietta, GA 30067, (800)825-0060.

2.   **ADIS Press.** Contact F. A. Davis Company, 1915 Arch Street, Philadelphia, PA 19103-9954, (215)568-2270.

3.   **Albert Whitman & Company.** 6340 Oakton Street, Morton Grove, IL 60053, (800)255-7675; (708)647-1355.

4.   **Alyson Publications.** Contact Inbrook Distribution Company, P.O. Box 120470, East Haven, CT 06512, (800)253-3605.

5.   **American Academy of Pediatrics.** Committee on Adolescence, Division of Publications, 131 Northwest Point Boulevard, P.O. Box 927, Elk Grove Village, IL 60009-0927, (800)433-9016.

6.   **American Film & Video.** 8901 Walden Road, Silver Spring, MD 20901, (800)78-VIDEO.

7.   **American Friends Service Committee.** 1501 Cherry Street, Philadelphia, PA 19102, (215)241-7048.

8.   **American Guidance Service.** Publishers Building, P.O. Box 99, Circle Pines, MN 55014-1796, (800)328-2560. In MN, call (800)247-5053.

9.   **Bantam Books.** 666 Fifth Avenue, New York, NY 10103, (800)223-6834.

10.   **Center for Early Adolescence.** University of North Carolina at Chapel Hill, Suite 211, Carr Mill Mall, Carrboro, NC 27510, (919)966-1148.

11.   **Center for Population Options.** 1025 Vermont Avenue NW, Washington, DC 20005, (202)347-5700.

12.   **Center on Human Policy.** School of Education, Syracuse University, 200 Huntington Hall, 2nd Floor, Syracuse, NY 13244-2340, (315)443-3851.

13.   **Channing L. Bete Company.** 200 State Road, South Deerfield, MA 01373, (413)665-7611.

14.   **Charles C. Thomas.** 2600 S. First Street, Springfield, IL 62794-9265, (217)789-8980.

15.   **College-Hill Press.** Contact Pro-Ed, 8700 Shoal Creek Boulevard, Austin, TX 78758, (512)451-3246.

16. **Columbia University Press.** 136 S. Broadway, Irvington-on Hudson, NY 10533, (914)591-9111.

17. **Council for Exceptional Children.** Division on Mental Retardation, 1920 Association Drive, Reston, VA 22091-1589, (703)620-3660.

18. **Crown Publishers.** c/o Harmony Books Division, 201 East 50th Street, New York, NY 10022, (212)751-2600.

19. **Ednick Communications.** Contact Pro-Ed, 8700 Shoal Creek Boulevard, Austin, TX 78758, (512)451-3246.

20. **Edwin Mellen Press.** P.O. Box 450, Lewiston, NY 14092, (716)754-2788.

21. **Family Life Education Associates.** P.O. Box 7466, Richmond, VA 23221, (804)264-5929.

22. **Federation for Children With Special Needs and the Center on Human Policy.** The Technical Assistance for Parent Programs (TAPP) Project, 312 Stuart Street, Second Floor, Boston, MA 02116, (617)482-2915.

23. **Gallaudet University.** Bookstore, 800 Florida Avenue NE, B20E, Washington, DC 20002-3695, (202)651-5380.

24. **Grune and Stratton.** c/o Prentice Hall, Attention: Mail Order Sales, 200 Old Tappan Road, Old Tappan, NJ 07675, (800)223-1360.

25. **Guilford Press.** 72 Spring Street, New York, NY 10012, (800)365-7006.

26. **Harcourt Brace Jovanovich.** 465 S. Lincoln Drive, Troy, MO 63379, (800)543-1918.

27. **Harper Collins.** Keystone Industrial Park, Reeves & Monahan, Scranton, PA 18512, (800)331-3761.

28. **Harrington Park Press.** 10 Alice Street, Binghamton, NY 13904-1580, (800)342-9678.

29. **Harvard University Press.** Attention: Customer Service, 79 Garden Street, Cambridge, MA 02138, (617)495-2600.

30. **Haworth Press.** 10 Alice Street, Binghamton, NY 13904-1580, (800)342-9678.

31. **Hazelden.** P.O. Box 176, Center City, MN 55012-0176, (800)328-9000.

32. **Hemisphere Publishing Corporation.** 1900 Frost Road, Suite 101, Bristol, PA 19007, (800)821-8312.

33. **International Diagnostic Services, Inc.** P.O. Box 389, Worthington, OH 43085, (614)885-2323.

34. **Interstate Research Associates.** Contact NICHCY, P.O. Box 1492, Washington, DC 20013, (800)695-0285.

35. **James Stanfield Publishing Company.** P.O. Box 41058, Santa Barbara, CA 93140, (800)421-6534.

36. **Johns Hopkins University Press.** 701 West 40th Street, Baltimore, MD 21211, (800)537-5487.

37. **MacMillan.** Front & Brown Streets, Riverside, NJ 08075, (800)257-5755.

38. **March of Dimes,** 1275 Mamaroneck Avenue, White Plains, NY 10605, (914)428-7100.

39. **National Association of School Psychologists.** Publications, 8455 Colesville Road, Silver Spring, MD 20910, (301)608-0500.

40. **National Association of Social Workers.** P.O. Box 92180, Washington, DC 20090-2180, (800)752-3590.

41. **National Center for Education in Maternal and Child Health.** 38th and R Street NW, Washington, DC 20057, (202)625-8400.

42. **National Center for Youth With Disabilities.** University of Minnesota, Box 721—UMHC, Harvard Street at East River Road, Minneapolis, MN 55455, (800)333-6293.

43. **National Down Syndrome Society.** 666 Broadway, New York, NY 10012, (800)221-4602.

44. **National Federation of the Blind.** 1800 Johnson Street, Baltimore, MD 21230, (301)659-9314.

45. **Network Publishing, Division of ETR Associates.** P.O. Box 1830, Santa Cruz, CA 95061-1830, (408)438-4060.

46. **Oregon Health Sciences University.** Child Development and Rehabilitation Center, P.O. Box 574, Portland, OR 97207, (503)494-7522.

47. **Paul H. Brookes Publishing Company.** P.O. Box 10624, Baltimore, MD 21285-0624, (800)638-3775.

48. **People Building Institute.** 330 Village Circle, Sheldon, IA 51201, (712)324-4873.

49. **Pergamon Press.** c/o MacMillan, Front & Brown Streets, Riverside, NJ 08075, (800)257-5755.

50. **Planned Parenthood Federation of America.** Marketing Department, 810 Seventh Avenue, New York, NY 10036, (212)819-9770. (This is the central headquarters for Planned Parenthood.)

51. **Plenum Publishing.** 233 Spring Street, New York, NY 10013-1578, (800)221-9369.

52. **Pro-Ed.** 8700 Shoal Creek Boulevard, Austin, TX 78758, (512)451-3246.

53. **Research Press.** 2612 North Mattis Avenue, Champaign, IL 61821, (217)352-3273.

54. **Robert E. Krieger Publishing.** P.O. Box 9542, Melbourne, FL 32902-9542, (407)724-9542.

55. **Bowker.** 121 Chanlon Road, New Providence, NJ 07974, (800)521-8110.

56. **Seal Press.** 3131 Western Avenue, No. 410, Seattle, WA 98121-1028, (206)283-7844.

57. **Seattle Rape Relief Crisis Center.** 1905 S. Jackson, Seattle, WA 98144, (206)325-5531.

58. **Seattle Rape Relief Developmental Disabilities Project.** 1905 S. Jackson, Seattle, WA 98144, (206)325-5531.

59. **Sex Information and Education Council of the U.S. (SIECUS).** 130 West 42nd Street, Suite 350, New York, NY 10003, (212)819-9770.

60. **Simon & Schuster.** Order Processing Department, P.O. Box 11071, Des Moines, IA 50336-1071, (515)284-6751.

61. **St. Martin's Press.** 175 Fifth Avenue, New York, NY 10010, (800)221-7945.

62. **St. Paul Ramsey Medical Center—HIHW.** 640 Jackson Street, St. Paul, MN 55101, (612)221-3569.

63. **United Cerebral Palsy Associations, Inc.** UCP/Lancaster County, 1811 Olde Homestead Lane, P.O. Box 10485, Lancaster, PA 17605-0485, (717)396-7965.

64. **Department of Health and Human Services.** Contact the Superintendent of Documents, U.S. Government Printing Office, Washington, DC 20402.

65. **Vida Publishing.** Primrose Lane/Highland Drive, P.O. Box 597, Mountville, PA 17554.

66. **Volcano Press.** P.O. Box 270, Volcano, CA 95689, (209)296-3445.

67. **Walker Publishing.** 720 Fifth Avenue, New York, NY 10019, (800)289-25537.

68. **Norton & Company.** c/o National Book Company, 800 Keystone Industrial Park, Scranton, PA 18512-4601, (800)223-2584.

69. **Young Adult Institute.** 460 West 34th Street, New York, NY 10001, (212)563-7474.

EDUCATIONAL TERMINOLOGY ASSOCIATED WITH SPECIAL EDUCATION

Ability Grouping—the grouping of children based on their achievement in an area of study.

Accelerated Learning—an educational process that allows students to progress through the curriculum at an increased pace.

Achievement—The level of a child's accomplishment on a test of knowledge or skill.

Adaptive Behavior—refers to an individual's social competence and ability to cope with the demands of the environment.

Adaptive Physical Education—a modified program of instruction implemented to meet the needs of special students.

Advocate—an individual, either a parent or professional, who attempts to establish or improve services for exceptional children.

Age Norms—standards based on the average performance of individuals in different age groups.

Agnosia—refers to the child's inability to recognize objects and their meaning, usually resulting from damage to the brain.

Amplification Device—any device that increases the volume of sound.

Anecdotal Record—a procedure for recording and analyzing observations of a child's behavior; an objective, narrative description.

Annual Goals—yearly activities or achievements, to be completed or attained by the disabled child, that are documented on the Individual Educational Plan.

Aphasia—the inability to acquire meaningful spoken language by the age of three, usually resulting from damage to or disease of the brain.

Articulation—the production of distinct language sounds by the vocal chords.

At Risk—usually refers to infants or children with a high potential for experiencing future medical or learning problems.

Attention Deficit Hyperactive Disorder (ADHD)—a psychiatric classification used to describe individuals who exhibit poor attention, distractibility, impulsivity, and hyperactivity.

Baseline Measure—the level or frequency of behavior prior to the implementation of an instructional procedure that will later be evaluated.

Behavior Modification—the techniques used to change behavior by applying principles of reinforcement learning.

Bilingual—having the ability to speak two languages.

Career Education—instruction that focuses on the application of skills and content area information necessary to cope with the problems of daily life, independent living, and vocational areas of interest.

Categorical Resource Room—an auxiliary pull-out program that offers supportive services to exceptional children with the same disability.

Cognition—the understanding of information.

Consultant Teacher—a supportive service for disabled children in which the services are provided by a specialist in the classroom.

Criterion-Referenced Tests—tests in which the child is evaluated on his or her own performance according to a set of criteria, and not in comparison with others.

Declassification—the process in which a disabled child is no longer considered in need of special education services. This requires a meeting of the CSE and can be requested by the parent, school, or child if over the age of 18.

Deficit—a level of performance that is less than expected for a child.

Desensitization—a technique used in reinforcement theory in which there is a weakening of a response, usually an emotional response.

Diagnosis—the specific disorder/s identified as a result of some evaluation.

Distractibility—difficulty in maintaining attention.

Due Process—the legal steps and processes outlined in educational law that protects the rights of disabled children.

Dysfluency—difficulty in the production of fluent speech, as in the example of stuttering.

Dyscalculia—a serious learning disability in which the child has an inability to calculate, apply, solve, or identify mathematical functions.

Dysorthographia—a serious learning disability that affects a child's ability to spell.

Dyslexia—a severe learning disability in which a child's ability to read is greatly impaired.

Dysgraphia—a serious learning disability in which the child has an inability or loss of ability to write.

Enrichment—providing a child with extra and more sophisticated learning experiences than those normally presented in the curriculum.

Exceptional Children—children whose school performance shows significant discrepancy between ability and achievement and who, as a result, require special instruction, assistance, or equipment.

Etiology—the cause of a problem.

Free Appropriate Public Education (FAPE)—used in PL94-142 to mean special education and related services that are provided at public expense and conform to the state requirements and the individual's IEP.

Group Home—a residential living arrangement for handicapped adults, especially the mentally retarded, along with several nonhandicapped supervisors.

Habilitation—an educational approach used with exceptional children that is directed toward the development of the necessary skills required for successful adulthood.

Homebound Instruction—a special education service in which teaching is provided by a specially trained instructor to students unable to attend school. A parent or guardian must always be present at the time of instruction. In some cases, the instruction may take place on a neutral site—not in the home or school.

Hyperactivity—behavior characterized by excessive motor activity or restlessness.

Impulsivity—nongoal-oriented activity exhibited by individuals who lack careful thought and reflection prior to a behavior.

Individualized Educational Plan—a written educational program that outlines a disabled child's current levels of performance, related services, educational goals, and modifications. This plan is developed by a team including the child's parent(s), teacher(s), and supportive staff.

Inclusion—returning disabled children to their home school so that they may be educated with nonhandicapped children in the same classroom.

Interdisciplinary Team—the collective efforts of individuals from a variety of disciplines in assessing the needs of a child.

Intervention—preventive, remedial, compensatory, or survival services made on behalf of a disabled individual.

Itinerant Teacher—a teacher hired by a school district to help in the education of a disabled child. The teacher is employed by an outside agency and may be responsible for several children in several districts.

Learning Disability—refers to children with average or above average potential intelligence who are experiencing a severe discrepancy between their ability and achievement.

Least Restrictive Environment—applies to the educational setting of exceptional children, and to the education of handicapped children with nonhandicapped children whenever realistic and possible. It is the least restrictive setting in which the disabled child can function without difficulty.

Mainstreaming—the practice of educating exceptional children in the regular classroom.

Mental Age—the level of intellectual functioning based on the average for children of the same chronological age. When dealing with severely disabled children, the mental age may be more reflective of levels of ability than the chronological age.

Mental Disability—refers to a disability in which the individual's intellectual level is measured within the subaverage range and there are marked impairments in social competence.

Native Language—the primary language used by an individual.

Noncategorical Resource Room—a resource room in regular school that provides services to children with all types of classified disabilities. The children with these disabilities are able to be maintained in a regular classroom.

Norm-Referenced Tests—tests used to compare a child's performance to the performance of others on the same measure.

Occupational Therapist—a professional who programs and delivers instructional activities and materials to help disabled children and adults participate in useful daily activities.

Paraprofessional—a trained assistant or parent who works with a classroom teacher in the education process.

Physical Therapist—a professional trained to help disabled individuals maintain and develop muscular and orthopedic capability and to make correct and useful movements.

PINS Petition—stands for "Person in Need of Supervision" and is a family court re[...] referral can be made by either the school or the parent and is usually made when a c[...] the age of 16 is out of control in terms of attendance, behavior, or some socially inappr[...] destructive pattern.

Positive Reinforcement—any stimulus or event that occurs after a behavior has been e[...] and that increases the possibility of that behavior occurring in the future.

Pupil Personnel Team—a group of professionals from the same school who meet on a regular basis to discuss children's problems and offer suggestions or a direction for resolution.

Pupils With Special Educational Needs (PSEN)—students defined as having math and reading achievement lower than the 23rd percentile and requiring remediation. These students are not considered disabled but are entitled to assistance to elevate their academic levels.

Pupil With Handicapping Condition (PHC)—refers to any child classified as disabled by the Committee on Special Education.

Related Services—services provided to disabled children to assist in their ability to learn and function in the least restrictive environment. Such services may include in-school counseling, speech and language services, and so on.

Remediation—an educational program designed to help children to overcome some deficit or disability through education and training.

Resource Room—an auxiliary service provided to disabled children for part of the school day. It is intended to service children's special needs so that they can be maintained within the least restrictive educational setting.

Screening—the process of examining groups of children in hopes of identifying potential high-risk children.

Section 504—refers to Section 504 of the Rehabilitation Act of 1973 in which guarantees are provided for the civil rights of disabled children and adults. It also applies to the provision of services for children whose disability is not severe enough to warrant classification, but who could benefit from supportive services and classroom modifications.

Self-Contained Class—a special classroom for exceptional children usually located within a regular school building.

Sheltered Workshop—a transitional or long-term work environment for disabled individuals who cannot work, or who are preparing for work in a regular setting. Within this setting, the individual can learn to perform meaningful, productive tasks and receive payment.

Surrogate Parent—a person other than the child's natural parent who has legal responsibility for the child's care and welfare.

Total Communication—the approach to the education of deaf students that combines oral speech, sign language, and finger spelling.

Token Economy—a system of reinforcing various behaviors through the delivery of tokens. These tokens can be in the form of stars, points, candy, chips, and so on.

Underachiever—a term generally used in reference to a child's lack of academic achievement in school. It is important, however, that the school identify the underlying causes of such underachievement, since it may be a symptom of a more serious problem.

Vocational Rehabilitation—a program designed to help disabled adults obtain and hold a job.

PSYCHOLOGICAL TERMINOLOGY ASSOCIATED WITH SPECIAL EDUCATION

Affective Reactions—psychotic reactions marked by extreme mood swings.

Anxiety—a general uneasiness of the mind characterized by irrational fears, panic, tension, and physical symptoms including palpitations, excessive sweating, and increased pulse rate.

Assessment—the process of gathering information about children in order to make educational decisions.

Baseline Data—an objective measure used to compare and evaluate the results obtained during some implementation of an instructional procedure.

Compulsion—a persistent, repetitive act that the individual cannot consciously control.

Confabulation—the act of replacing memory loss by fantasy or by some reality that is not true for the occasion.

Defense Mechanisms—the unconscious means by which an individual protects himself or herself against impulses or emotions that are too uncomfortable or threatening. Examples of these mechanisms include the following.

    Denial—a defense mechanism in which the individual refuses to admit the reality of some unpleasant event, situation, or emotion.

    Displacement—the disguising of the goal or intention of a motive by substituting another in its place.

    Intellectualization—a defense mechanism in which the individual exhibits anxious or moody deliberation, usually about abstract matters.

    Projection—the disguising of a source of conflict by displacing one's own motives to someone else.

    Rationalization—the interpretation of one's own behavior to conceal the motive it expresses by assigning the behavior to another motive.

    Reaction Formation—a complete disguise of a motive expressed in a form that is directly opposite to its original intent.

    Repression—the psychological process involved in not permitting memories and motives to enter consciousness, even though they are operating at an unconscious level.

    Supression—the act of consciously inhibiting an impulse, affect, or idea, as in the deliberate act of forgetting something in order not to have to think about it.

Delusion—a groundless, irrational belief or thought, usually of grandeur or of persecution. It is usually a characteristic of paranoia.

Depersonalization—a nonspecific syndrome in which the individual senses that he or she has lost personal identity, that he or she is different, strange, or not real.

Echolalia—the repetition of what other people say as if echoing them.

Etiology—refers to the cause or causes of something.

Hallucination—an image (visual, aural, etc.) that is not real but is regarded as a real sensory experience by the person.

Magical Thinking—refers to primitive and prelogical thinking in which the child creates an outcome to meet a fantasy rather than the reality.

Neologisms—made-up words that have meaning only to the child or adult.

Obsession—a repetitive and persistent idea that intrudes into a person's thoughts.

Panic Attack—a serious episode of anxiety in which the individual experiences a variety of symptoms including palpitations, dizziness, nausea, chest pains, trembling, fear of dying, and fear of losing control. These symptoms are not the result of any medical cause.

Paranoia—a personality disorder in which the individual exhibits extreme suspiciousness of the motives of others.

Phobia—an intense irrational fear, usually acquired through conditioning to an unpleasant object or event.

Projective Tests—methods used by psychologists and psychiatrists to study personality dynamics through a series of structured or ambiguous stimuli.

Psychosis—a serious mental disorder in which the individual has difficulty differentiating between fantasy and reality.

Rorschach Test—an unstructured psychological test in which the individual is asked to project responses to a series of ten inkblots.

School Phobia—a form of separation anxiety in which the child's concerns and anxieties are centered around school issues and as a result he or she has an extreme fear about going to school.

Symptom—any sign, physical or mental, that stands for something else. Symptoms are usually generated from the tension of conflicts. The more serious the problem or conflict, the more frequent and intense the symptom.

Syndrome—a group of symptoms.

Thematic Apperception Test—a structured psychological test in which the individual is asked to project his or her feelings onto a series of drawings or photos.

Wechsler Scales of Intelligence—a series of individual intelligence tests measuring global intelligence through a variety of subtests.

MEDICAL TERMINOLOGY ASSOCIATED WITH SPECIAL EDUCATION

Albinism—a congenital condition marked by severe deficiency in or total lack of pigmentation.

Amblyopia—a dimness of sight without any indication of change in the eye's structure.

Amniocentesis—a medical procedure done during the early stages of pregnancy for the purpose of identifying certain genetic disorders in the fetus.

Anomaly—some irregularity in development, or a deviation from the standard.

Anoxia—a lack of oxygen.

Aphasia—the inability to acquire meaningful spoken language by the age of 3 as a result of brain damage.

Apraxia—pertains to problems with voluntary, or purposeful, muscular movement with no evidence of motor impairment.

Astigmatism—a visual defect resulting in blurred vision, caused by uneven curvature of the cornea or lens. The condition is usually corrected by lenses.

Ataxia—a form of cerebral palsy in which the individual suffers from a loss of muscle coordination, especially those movements relating to balance and position.

Athetosis—a form of cerebral palsy characterized by involuntary, jerky, purposeless, and repetitive movements of the extremities, head, and tongue.

Atrophy—degeneration of tissue.

Audiogram—a graphic representation of the results of a hearing test.

Audiologist—a specialist trained in the evaluation and remediation of auditory disorders.

Binocular Vision—vision using both eyes working together to perceive a single image.

Blind, Legally—visual acuity measured at 20/200 in the better eye with best correction of glasses or contact lenses. Vision measured at 20/200 means the individual must be 20 feet from something to be able to see what the normal eye can see at 200 feet.

Cataract—a condition of the eye in which the crystalline lens becomes cloudy or opaque. As a result, a reduction or loss of vision occurs.

Catheter—a tube inserted into the body to allow for injections or withdrawal of fluids, or to maintain an opening in a passageway.

Cerebral Palsy—an abnormal succession of human movement or motor functioning resulting from a defect, insult to, or disease of the central nervous system.

Conductive Hearing Loss—a hearing loss resulting from obstructions in the outer or middle ear or some malformations that interfere in the conduction of sound waves to the inner ear. This condition may be corrected medically or surgically.

Congenital—present at birth.

Cretinism—a congenital condition associated with a thyroid deficiency that can result in stunted physical growth and mental retardation.

Cyanosis—a lack of oxygen in the blood characterized by a blue discoloration of the skin.

Cystic Fibrosis—an inherited disorder affecting pancreas, salivary, mucous, and sweat glands that causes severe, long-term respiratory difficulties.

Diplegia—paralysis that affects either both arms or both legs.

Down Syndrome—a medical abnormality caused by a chromosomal anomaly that often results in moderate to severe mental retardation. The child with Down Syndrome will exhibit certain physical characteristics such as a large tongue, heart problems, poor muscle tone, and broad, flat bridge of the nose.

Electroencephalogram (EEG)—a graphic representation of the electrical output of the brain.

Encopresis—a lack of bowel control that may also have psychological causes.

Endogenous—originating from within.

Enureusis—a lack of bladder control that may also have psychological causes.

Exogenous—originating from external causes.

Fetal Alcohol Syndrome—a condition usually found in the infants of alcoholic mothers. As a result, low birth weight, severe retardation, and cardiac, limb, and other physical defects may be present.

Field of Vision—the area of space visible with both eyes while looking straight ahead; measured in degrees.

Glaucoma—an eye disease characterized by excessively high pressure inside the eyeball. If untreated, the condition can result in total blindness.

Grand Mal Seizure—the most serious and severe form of an epileptic seizure in which the individual exhibits violent convulsions, loses consciousness, and becomes rigid.

Hemiplegia—paralysis involving the extremities on the same side of the body.

Hemophilia—an inherited deficiency in the blood clotting factor that can result in serious internal bleeding.

Hertz—a unit of sound frequency used to measure pitch.

Hydrocephalus—a condition present at birth or developing soon afterward from excess cerebrospinal fluid in the brain; results in an enlargement of the head and mental retardation. This condition is sometimes prevented by the surgical placement of a shunt, which allows for the proper drainage of the built-up fluids.

Hyperactivity—excessive physical and muscular activity characterized by extreme inattention, excessive restlessness, and mobility. The condition is usually associated with Attention Deficit Disorder or learning disabilities.

Hyperopia—farsightedness; a condition causing difficulty with seeing near objects.

Hypertonicity—heightened state of muscle tension.

Hypotonicity—an inability to maintain muscle tone, or an inability to maintain muscle tension, or resistance to stretch.

Insulin—a protein hormone produced by the pancreas that regulates carbohydrate metabolism.

Iris—the opaque, colored portion of the eye.

Juvenile Diabetes—a children's disease characterized by an inadequate secretion or use of insulin resulting in excessive sugar in the blood and urine. This condition is usually controlled by diet and/or medication. In certain cases, however, control may be difficult and if untreated, serious complications may arise such as visual impairments, limb amputation, coma, and death.

Meningitis—an inflammation of the membranes covering the brain and spinal cord. If untreated, can result in serious complications.

Meningocele—a type of spina bifida in which there is protrusion of the covering of the spinal cord through an opening in the vertebrae.

Microcephaly—a disorder involving the cranial cavity characterized by the development of a small head. Retardation usually occurs from the lack of space for brain development.

Monoplegia—paralysis of a single limb.

Multiple Sclerosis—a progressive deterioration of the protective sheath surrounding the nerves leading to a degeneration and failure of the body's central nervous system.

Muscular Dystrophy—a group of diseases that eventually weakens and destroys muscle tissue, leading to a progressive deterioration of the body.

Myopia—nearsightedness; a condition that results in blurred vision for distance objects.

Neonatal—the time usually associated with the period between the onset of labor and six weeks following birth.

Neurologically Impaired—exhibiting problems associated with the functioning of the central nervous system.

Nystagmus—a rapid, rhythmic, and involuntary movement of the eyes. This condition may result in difficulty reading or fixating on objects.

Ocular Mobility—refers to the eye's ability to move.

Ophthalmologist—a medical doctor trained to deal with diseases and conditions of the eye.

Optometrist—a professional trained to examine eyes for defects and prescribe corrective lenses.

Optic Nerve—the nerve in the eye that carries impulses to the brain.

Optician—a specialist trained to grind lenses according to a prescription.

Ossicles—the three small bones of the ear that transmit sound waves to the eardrum. They consist of the malleus, incus, and stapes.

Osteogenesis Imperfecta—also known as "brittle bone disease," this hereditary condition affects the growth of bones and causes them to break easily.

Otitis Media—Middle ear infection.

Otolaryngologist—a medical doctor specializing in diseases of the ear and throat.

Otologist—a medical doctor specializing in the diseases of the ear.

Otosclerosis—a bony growth in the middle ear that develops around the base of the stapes, impeding its movement and causing hearing loss.

Organic—factors usually associated with the central nervous system that cause a handicapping condition.

Paralysis—an impairment to or a loss of voluntary movement or sensation.

Paraplegia—a paralysis usually involving the lower half of the body, including both legs, as a result of injury to or disease of the spinal cord.

Perinatal—occurring at or immediately following birth.

Petit Mal Seizure—a mild form of epilepsy characterized by dizziness and momentary lapses of consciousness.

Phenylketonuria—referred to as PKU; this inherited metabolic disease usually results in severe retardation. If detected at birth, however, a special diet can reduce the serious complications associated with the condition.

Photophobia—an extreme sensitivity of the eyes to light. This condition is common in albino children.

Postnatal—occurring after birth.

Prenatal—occurring before birth.

Prosthesis—an artificial device used to replace a missing body part.

Psychomotor Seizure—epileptic seizure in which the individual exhibits many automatic seizure activities of which he or she is not aware.

Pupil—the opening in the middle of the iris that expands and contracts to let in light.

Quadriplegia—paralysis involving all four limbs.

Retina—the back portion of the eye, containing nerve fibers that connect to the optic nerve on which the image is focused.

Retinitis Pigmentosa—a degenerative eye disease in which the retina gradually atrophies, causing a narrowing of the field of vision.

Retrolental Fibroplasia—an eye disorder resulting from excessive oxygen in incubators of premature babies.

Rh Incompatibility—a blood condition in which the fetus has Rh positive blood and the mother has Rh negative blood, leading to a buildup of antibodies that attack the fetus. If untreated, can result in birth defects.

Rheumatic Fever—a disease characterized by acute inflammation of the joints, fever, skin rash, nosebleeds, and abdominal pain. This disease often damages the heart by scarring its tissues and valves.

Rigidity Cerebral Palsy—a type of cerebral palsy characterized by minimal muscle elasticity, and little or no stretch reflex, which creates stiffness.

Rubella—referred to as German measles, this communicable disease is usually only of concern when developed by women during the early stages of pregnancy. If contracted at that time, there is a high probability of severe handicaps in the offspring.

Sclera—the tough white outer layer of the eyeball that protects as well as holds structure in place.

Scoliosis—a weakness of the muscles that results in a serious abnormal curvature of the spine. This condition may be corrected with surgery or a brace.

Semicircular Canals—the three canals within the middle ear that are responsible for maintaining balance.

Sensorineural Hearing Loss—a hearing disorder resulting from damage or dysfunction of the cochlea.

Shunt—a tube that is inserted into the body to drain fluid from one part to another. This procedure is common in cases of hydrocephalus to remove excessive cerebrospinal fluid from the head and redirect it to the heart or intestines.

Spasticity—a type of cerebral palsy characterized by tense, contracted muscles, resulting in muscular incoordination.

Spina Bifida Occulta—a type of spina bifida characterized by a protrusion of the spinal cord and membranes. This form of the condition does not always cause serious disability.

Strabismus—crossed eyes.

Tremor—a type of cerebral palsy characterized by consistent, strong, uncontrolled movements.

Triplegia—paralysis of three of the body's limbs.

Usher's Syndrome—an inherited combination of visual and hearing impairments.

Visual Acuity—sharpness or clearness of vision.

Vitreous Humor—the jellylike fluid that fills most of the interior of the eyeball.

TERMINOLOGY ASSOCIATED WITH OCCUPATIONAL THERAPY

Abduction—movement of limb outward, away from body.

Active Movements—movements a child does without help.

Adaptive Equipment—devices used to position or to teach special skills.

Asymmetrical—one side of the body different from the other—unequal or dissimilar.

Associated Reactions—increase of stiffness in spastic arms and legs resulting from effort.

Ataxic—no balance, jerky.

Athetosis—uncontrolled and continuously unwanted movements.

Atrophy—wasting of the muscles.

Automatic Movements—necessary movements done without thought or effort.

Balance—not falling over, ability to keep a steady position.

Bilateral Motor—refers to skill and performance in purposeful movement that requires interaction between both sides of the body in a smooth manner.

Clonus—shaky movements of spastic muscle.

Compensory Movement—a form of movement that is atypical in relation to normal patterns of movement.

Congenital—from birth.

Coordination—combination of muscle in movement.

Contracture—permanently tight muscle or joint.

Crossing the Midline—refers to skill and performance in crossing the vertical midline of the body.

Deformity—body or limb fixed in abnormal position.

Diplegia—legs mostly affected.

Distractable—not able to concentrate.

Equilibrium—balance.

Equilibrium Reactions—automatic patterns of body movements that enable restoration and maintenance of balance against gravity.

Equinus—toe walks.

Extension—straightening of the trunk and limbs.

Eye-Hand Coordination—eye is used as a tool for directing the hand to perform efficiently.

Facilitation—making it possible for the child to move.

Figure-Ground Perception—ability to see foreground against the background.

Fine Motor—small muscle movements, use of hands and fingers.

Flexion—bending of elbows, hips, knees, etc.

Fluctuating Tone—changing from one degree of tension to another, for example, from low to high tone.

Form Constancy—ability to perceive an object as possessing invariant properties such as shape, size, color, and brightness.

Swing to Gait—walking with crutches or walker by moving crutches forward and swinging body up to crutches.

Swing Thru—walking with crutches by moving crutches forward and swinging body in front of the crutches.

Genu Valgus—knocked knee.

Genu Varum—bowlegged.

Gross Motor—coordinated movements of all parts of the body for performance.

Guarding Techniques—techniques used to help students maintain balance including contact guarding, when a student requires hands-on contact to maintain balance.

Guarded Supervision—an individual is close to the student to provide physical support if balance is lost while sitting, standing, or walking.

Head Control—ability to control the position of the head.

Hemiplegia—one side of the body affected.

Hypertonicity—increased muscle tone.

Hypotonicity—decreased muscle tone.

Inhibition—positions and movements that stop muscle tightness.

Involuntary Movements—unintended movements.

Kyphosis—increased rounding of the upper back.

Lordosis—sway back or increased curve in the back.

Manual Muscle Test—test of isolated muscle strength:

normal	-	100%
good	-	80%
fair	-	50%
poor	-	20%
zero	-	0%

Mobility—movement of a body muscle or body part, or movement of the whole body from one place to another.

Motivation—making the student want to move or perform.

Motor Planning—ways in which the body and limbs work together to make movement, also known as praxis.

Nystagmus—series of automatic back-and-forth eye movements.

Organization—a student's ability to organize himself or herself in approach to and performance of activities.

Orthosis—brace.

Paraplegia—paralysis of the lower half of the body with involvement of both legs.

Passive—anything that is done to the student without his or her help or cooperation.

Pathological—due to or involving abnormality.

Perception—the organization of sensation from useful functioning.

Perservation—unnecessary repetition of speech or movement.

Positioning—ways of placing an individual that will help normalize postural tone and facilitate normal patterns of movement, and that may involve the use of adaptive equipment.

Position in Space—child's ability to understand the relationship of an object to himself or herself.

Postural Balance—skill and performance in developing and maintaining body posture while sitting, standing, or engaging in an activity.

Praxis—ability to think through a new task that requires movement, also known as motor planning.

Pronation—turning of the hand with palm down.

Prone—lying on the stomach.

Quadriplegia—whole body affected.

Range of Motion—joint motion.

Reflex—stereotypic posture and movement that occurs in relation to specific eliciting stimuli and outside of conscious control.

Righting Reactions—ability to put head and body right when positions are abnormal or uncomfortable.

Right/Left Discrimination—skill and performance in differentiating right from left and vice versa.

Rigidity—very stiff movements and postures.

Rotation—movement of the trunk; the shoulders move opposite to the hips.

Sensation—feeling.

Sensory-Motor Experience—the feeling of one's own movements.

Sequencing—the ordering of visual patterns in time and space.

Scoliosis—C or S curvature of the spine.

Spasm—sudden tightness of muscles.

Spasticity—increased muscle tone.

Spatial Relations—ability to perceive the position of two or more objects in relation to self and to each other.

Stair Climbing—methods of climbing include mark stepping—ascending or descending stairs one step at a time, and alternating steps—step over step.

Stereognosis—the identification of form and nature of object through the sense of touch.

Subluxation—a partial dislocation where joint surfaces remain in contact with one another.

Supination—turning of hand with palm up.

Symmetrical—both sides equal.

Tactile—pertaining to the sense of touch.

Tandem Walking—walks in a forward progression, placing heel to toe.

Tone—firmness of muscles.

Vestibular System—a sensory system that responds to the position of the head in relation to gravity and accelerated and decelerated movements.

Visual Memory—ability to recall visual stimuli, in terms of form, detail, position, and other significant features on both short- and long-term basis.

Visual-Motor Integration—the ability to combine visual input with purposeful voluntary movement of the hand and other body parts involved in the activity.

Voluntary Movements—movements done with attention and with concentration.

Appendix L

ABBREVIATIONS ASSOCIATED WITH SPECIAL EDUCATION

ACLC—Assessment of Children's Language Comprehension

ADHD—Attention Deficit Hyperactive Disorder

AE—Age Equivalent

AUD.DIS—Auditory Discrimination

BINET—Stanford Binet Intelligence Test

BVMGT—Bender Visual Motor Gestalt Test

CA—Chronological Age

CAT—Childrens Apperception Test

CEC—Council for Exceptional Children

CP—Cerebral Palsy

CSE—Committee on Special Education

DAP—Draw a Person Test

dB—Decibel—Hearing Measurement

DDST—Denver Developmental Screening Test

DQ—Developmental Quotient

DTLA-3—Detroit Tests of Learning Aptitude-3

ED—Emotionally Disturbed

EMR—Educable Mentally Retarded

FAPE—Free Appropriate Public Education

fq—Frequency Range—Hearing Measurement

GE—Grade Equivalent

GFW—Goldman-Fristoe-Woodcock Test of Auditory Discrimination

HH—Hard of Hearing

HTP—House-Tree-Person Test

Hz—Hertz—Hearing Measurement

IEU—Intermediate Educational Unit

IHE—Institutions of Higher Education

IQ—Intelligence Quotient

ITPA—Illinois Tests of Psycholinguistic Abilities

LA—Learning Aptitude

LD—Learning Disabled

LEA—Local Education Agency

LPR—Local Percentile Rank

MA—Mental Age

MBD—Minimal Brain Dysfunction

MH—Multiply Handicapped

MMPI—Minnesota Multiphasic Personality Inventory

MR—Mentally Retarded

MVPT—Motor-Free Visual Perception Test

NPR—National Percentile Rank

PHC—Pupils With Handicapping Conditions

PIAT—Peabody Individual Achievement Test

PINS—Person in Need of Supervision

PLA—Psycholinguistic Age

PQ—Perceptual Quotient

PPVT—Peabody Picture Vocabulary Test

PR—Percentile Rank

PS—Partially Sighted

PSEN—Pupils With Special Educational Needs

PTA—Pure Tone Average—Hearing Measurement

SAI—School Abilities Index

SCSIT—Southern California Sensory Integration Tests

SEA—State Education Agency

SIT—Slosson Intelligence Test

SRT—Speech Reception Threshhold—Hearing Measurement

TACL—Test for Auditory Comprehension of Language

TAT—Thematic Apperception Test

TMR—Trainable Mentally Retarded

TOWL—Test of Written Language

TWS—Larsen-Hammill Test of Written Spelling

VAKT—Visual/Auditory/Kinesthetic/Tactile

VIS.DIS—Visual Discrimination

VMI—Beery-Buktenica Developmental Test of Visual Motor Integration

WAIS-R—Wechsler Adult Intelligence Scale-Revised

WISC-R—Wechsler Intelligence Scale for Children-Revised

WISC-III—Wechsler Intelligence Scale for Children-III

WPPSI-R—Wechsler Preschool and Primary Scale of Intelligence-Revised

WRAT-R—Wide Range Achievement Test-Revised

INDEX

Y